TOTAL BODY

TRANSFORMATION

SECRETS

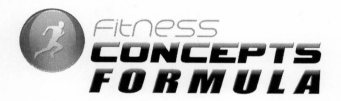

DR. SAMAN BAKHTIAR DC

DISCLAIMER AND TERMS OF USE AGREEMENT

The author and publisher have used their best efforts in preparing this report. The author and publisher make no representation or warranties with respect to the accuracy, applicability, fitness, or completeness of the contents of this report. The information contained in this report is strictly for educational purposes. Therefore, if you wish to apply ideas contained in this report, you are taking full responsibility for your actions.

Every effort has been made to accurately represent this product and its potential. However, there is no guarantee that you will improve in any way using the techniques and ideas in these materials. Examples in these materials are not to be interpreted as a promise or guarantee of anything. Self-help and improvement potential is entirely dependent on the person using our product, ideas and techniques.

Your level of improvement in attaining the results claimed in our materials depends on the time you devote to the program, ideas and techniques mentioned, along with your knowledge and various skills. Since these factors differ according to individuals, we cannot guarantee your success or improvement level. Nor are we responsible for any of your actions.

Many factors will be important in determining your actual results, and no guarantees are made that you will achieve results similar to ours or anybody else's; in fact no guarantees are made that you will achieve any results from our ideas and techniques in our material.

The author and publisher disclaim any warranties (express or implied), merchantability, or fitness for any particular purpose. The author and publisher shall in no event be held liable to any party for any direct, indirect, punitive, special, incidental or other consequential damages arising directly or indirectly from any use of this material, which is provided "as is," and without warranties.

As always, the advice of a competent professional should be sought.

The author and publisher do not warrant the performance, effectiveness or applicability of any sites listed or linked to in this report.

All links are for information purposes only and are not warranted for content, accuracy or any other implied or explicit purpose.

PREFACE

I want to dedicate this book first and foremost to God, as without his blessings, none of us would be here today.

I also want to dedicate this book to my super-woman mother, Sheida Bakhtiar. She is the strongest woman that I have ever met. When I say strong, I don't mean physically strong, as she is 4'11" and weighs about 105lb.

Strong here means raising a boy as a single parent, working full-time, sending me to the best schools, and bringing us all the way to America for a better life and opportunity.

Thank you, mother, for teaching me the value of hard work and perseverance. You are truly a SUPER WOMAN.

I also want to dedicate this book to my beautiful wife, Johnette. She is truly the most beautiful woman, not only on the outside but inside as well. Johentte, thank you for believing in me when I didn't even believe in myself.

I also want to dedicate this book to my new love: my beautiful baby girl, Bailee, who was born on July 3rd, 2009. She has truly given me a whole new meaning to life. I love you dearly.

I also want to thank the countless others who have had a huge impact on my life. That is a whole new book by itself.

Before we get started, a little history and background is necessary to understand the why's, how's and who's of this book.

As a young boy who was born and raised in Tehran, Iran, I played soccer (a.k.a. football) every chance that I got.

I mean, I was obsessed with soccer. I had a soccer ball with me everywhere that I went.

I drove the neighbors crazy because all they heard was the pounding of the soccer ball all day and night in the neighborhood.

I will never forget the day when I was 7 years old and I met all the players from my favorite Persian team, the Perspolis.

I took pictures with them and even went to their locker room.

I then aspired to be just like them and wanted to do nothing but become the best soccer player ever. I played, watched and breathed soccer 24/7.

Unfortunately, the war started getting really bad between Iran and Iraq, and having Bakhtiar as a last name wasn't helping me at all. (Those of you who know history really well likely already know that my great uncle, Shapour Bakhtiar, was the Prime Minister of Iran before the revolution.)

My mom decided it would be best for us to leave the country and move abroad. (That is a whole new book by itself also.)

We lived in France for one year and then finally, in 1985, moved to the United States.

We moved to a small town in Pennsylvania called Sharon, since my uncle - the only relative that we had in the U.S. - lived there. (He moved there to attend and graduate from Youngstown State University.)

My uncle Ali was gracious enough to take us in and let us stay with him until we got our own place.

My uncle Ali is truly one of the most genuine, generous people in this whole world. He still lives in Sharon with his wife, Beth, and his 5 beautiful children: Shannon, Brian, Reza, Kiley and Ellie.

When I got to Sharon in 1985, I had my soccer ball (which I knew as a football) and was happily kicking it around the neighborhood, but there was one problem: their football and my football were totally different.

Their ball wasn't even round and didn't really have anything to do with the foot.

As I started 7th grade in Sharon High School, no one knew the sport that I called football (known as soccer here in the U.S.). They didn't even have a soccer team.

After school, my mom picked me up and dropped me off at the Buhl Club, where most of the town folk went to play various sports and recreation.

I started playing a little basketball and working out with some machine weights.

Then I had a brilliant idea. In 9th grade, I was going to try out for the basketball team. All of a sudden, I started to feel like I was a star again. Since I couldn't be a soccer star, I decided to become a basketball star.

I will never forget the day of the 9th grade basketball tryouts. I was ready; I had my new converse 76ers shoes and new socks, and I was ready to be a star.

We practiced all weekend and the coach was going to announce by the end of practice Sunday who made the team.

It was a cold Sunday morning with at least a foot of snow on the ground. We all sat nervously on the bleachers as the coach arrived and called out names of the kids who made the team.

I was devastated when my name wasn't called, which meant that I didn't make the team.

I didn't show any emotions in front of other kids, but I remember walking back to my uncle's house on the other side of town, through a foot of snow, while crying my eyes out.

It was truly a day that I will never forget. Later, when my Mom came home and saw my face, she immediately knew what had happened.

She comforted me and gave me a speech that I will never forget.

She said "Son, you can do anything that you put your mind to. All you need to do is work hard and persevere. Never give up." She also went on to tell me, "When you were child and fell down, you always looked at me and cried to pick you up. Guess what, son, I didn't pick you up because I wanted you to learn to stand on your own two feet and learn to persevere."

With her words of encouragement fresh in my mind, I started going back to the Buhl Club. I tell you, it wasn't easy, especially being a minority in Sharon, Pennsylvania.

Kids being how they are, they made fun of me for not making the team. They also made racial remarks about me since I was pretty much the only non-American in Sharon High School at that time.

I paid them no attention and went on to keep playing basketball. I also started hitting the weights.

After a few months of working out, everyone started noticing the changes in my arms and my chest, and they started asking me questions.

Flattered by all of the attention, I immediately fell in love with weight training and directed all my focus to learning as much as I could about training, nutrition, and supplements.

And the rest is history.......

Between the years of 1992-1996, I competed in bodybuilding competitions, winning the Tri-State teenage competition, all while attending Penn State University full-time. I also worked as a bouncer at a local bar in State College called "The Boogie", thanks to my very good friend Fred Sahakian, who gave me that opportunity. Fred was also the owner of Body Works Gym in State College,

In 1996, I moved to Irvine, California, to live with my uncle and aunt all while attending the Los Angeles College of Chiropractic.

Although my uncle and aunt lived in a very small 2-bedroom apartment, they both welcomed me with open arms and allowed me to stay in their spare bedroom.

Thank you, Uncle Amir and Aunt Farah, for opening your house to me.

While I attended Chiropractic school, I competed in and won the Mr. Orange County Bantamweight class in 1999.

In December of 1999, I graduated with a Doctorate degree of Chiropractic and started Fitness Concepts.

From 1999-2005, I grew Fitness Concepts to one of the top personal training centers in the country, all while competing and winning the following bodybuilding titles in 5 different weight classes (something never before done by anyone):

1)   Mr. Orange County

2)   Mr. San Diego

3)   Mr. Pittsburgh

4)   Mr. Los Angeles

5)   Emerald Cup

6)   Runner up Mr. USA

I am not stating that to impress you, but I am trying to impress upon you that you can have a nice physique even if you're busy. It takes a little discipline, and special attention must be paid to time management. But it can be definitely done.

Have you heard the old saying, "If you want something done, give it to a busy person"?

How many people do you know who don't do anything day after day, yet can't seem to get the smallest task done?

Consider if you worked out 5 hours/week. That's only 3% of your overall time each week.

As I mentioned earlier, I have a beautiful wife, a beautiful daughter, and a few successful businesses that I have to nurture.

Are you starting to see my point? If not, let me explain something to you. Life is not going to stop because you want to get in shape.

There are always things that are going to "come up" and make it difficult for you to work out and take care of your health and your business. That's just life, no matter if you are a blue collar worker or the CEO of a fortune 500 company.

Until you start to make your health and fitness a top priority, everything else is going to get in the way.

This book is for people who want to have a balanced life, people who want to take care of their health and fitness without giving up their careers and spending so much time away from their spouse that they end up divorced and lonely.

Consider this: Ever since I was 14, I have worked, gone to school, started my own business, got married, had a baby, started a few businesses, and still managed to maintain a decent physique.

So, this book is dedicated to busy individuals who are striving to maintain their health and fitness all while "taking care of business."

I want you to know that no matter your current condition, you can still:

1) Get in shape

2) Maintain your shape

3) Have more energy

4) Have better self esteem

5) Feel and look "hot" or "sexy"

6) Get healthy

TABLE OF CONTENTS

INTRODUCTION

Thank you so much for taking the time to read this book, which has all of the information you need to really change the way you look at exercise and nutrition programs. The information on these pages will show you exactly how I have helped thousands of my clients get in the best shape of their lives.

This book basically covers everything I've learned during eighteen years as a top national competitive bodybuilder and one of the most sought-after fitness professionals. There are usually two different types of people in the fitness industry. You have people who know what to do because they've done it. These people are usually "meat heads" or "Gym rats" that know what to do but can't explain why or how it works. You then have people who studied everything about working out and nutrition but don't have a clue as to real-world application. They have never actually been in the "trenches". I, on the other hand, did both. I was the nerd and the body builder. So, actually, I'm the one who went to school, learned a fitness concept, and then, after school, ran to the gym and applied it. So I'm here to teach you what really works in the real world. I will try to put everything in layman terms for you to understand, even if you're a beginner, so you can apply these concepts to get the results that you want: getting and staying healthy forever. While anybody can all of a

FITNESS CONCEPTS FORMULA

sudden lose a bunch of weight, gain it back, and go through that vicious yo-yo cycle; the art of losing weight long-term is to lose the fat and keep the muscle.

So, first things first. The first thing that you need to do is to sit down and set specific goals. I want you to write down your goal right now; be as specific as possible. For example, maybe you want to weight 172 lbs, have a 29-inch waist, or reach a body fat of 24%. Specific. The last thing you want to say is, "I want to lose a few pounds," which is not a measurable goal – so you'll never know the amazing feeling when you reach your goal.

Now, the next step is to put your goal in writing, and I want you to look at it every day, preferably in the morning. Be obsessed about it; look at it as often as possible. The more you look at your goal, the more it is going to settle into your subconscious mind, and the more you are going to act on it. If your goal does not have anything to do with your body shape or weight, then say how you want to feel.

Here is something that I do with my clients that works like a charm:

I have them write a short-term, medium-term and long–term goal. Short-term is anywhere between 6-12 weeks, medium-term is between 24-36 weeks, and long-term is anywhere between 12-24 months.

Each goal is then assigned a hard deadline.

The goal has to be very specific and measurable.

Then I will have them write down obstacles that might prevent them from reaching their goals, followed by writing down what needs to be done to overcome the obstacles.

They write down the rewards for when they reach that goal.

They write down the punishment for not reaching that goal.

They decide who will be the "referee" for keeping them accountable.

When you set a goal, it's very important that you guard that goal and do everything in your power to achieve it. Not achieving a goal IS NOT OK.

By setting a goal and not achieving it, you are telling yourself that it's OK to break promises to yourself. After all, isn't a goal a promise to yourself?

I want to share something about me that not many people know. In 1996, during my senior year at Penn State, I decided to get ready for the Mr. Pittsburgh contest. I trained hard and was very strict on my diet. Two weeks before the contest, I cheated on my diet. I was devastated because I thought that I had ruined everything.

I kept having negative self talk and told myself things like, "Sam you are a loser," and "If you can't stick to your diet, then you don't deserve to be a bodybuilder." So I decided to drop out of the contest and ate nothing but pizza and donuts for two weeks.

I decided to go to the contest as a spectator after eating crap for two weeks. When I watched the show from the stands, I discovered that I would have won the contest even AFTER eating crap for two weeks.

The only person that beat me was me, and no one else. That situation taught me a couple of huge lessons that I was able to apply to my career later on to win a first place title in every weight class. To this date, I don't know of anyone else accomplishing this

Here are the lessons that I learned:

1) Don't worry about winning every battle. Focus on winning the war.

2) Loosing feels 100x worse when you self-defeat. Never doubt yourself; just go for it.

3) Don't make your diet too complicated and end up driving yourself crazy. Keep it simple.

You see, everybody wants to look good but nobody wants to do the work. Remember Ronnie Coleman's famous words in his video as he was lifting 800 lbs? He said, "Everyone wants to be a bodybuilder but no one wants to lift these heavy-ass weights." I tell my clients all the time that "You can't out-train a bad diet." I remember when I talked to the legendary Sugar Shane Mosely, one of the boxing all-time greatest. He said, "Everybody wanted to be a fighter until they get hit." You see, there are always some sacrifices if you want to achieve anything in life. Set your goals big. Set your sights high. You can achieve what you want to achieve. There's no reason you should say, "Oh, I'm not going to be able to do all that," or "Oh, I'm 58; I could never look like that." No, you can. I have seen it happen. I have people in my gym right now who are 61 years old and in the best shape of the lives ever. Better than they were in their 20's, even. So that can happen. So don't delay with your own "Oh" statement. Don't set up an excuse and say you can't this or you can't do that. Don't let anybody tell you that. You can achieve what you set your mind to.

When I graduated from high school, I weighed 129 pounds. People questioned, "You are going to be a body builder? Really? *You?*" Yet I went on to become the first body builder in history to win a first place title in every weight class. If I had listened to the people who had doubted me, then I would not have won those titles.

But I must say, your goals must have realistic deadlines. Every other week, I have somebody coming into my office and delcaring, "Sam I'm going on a cruise, and I need to lose 30 pounds by next week." Not gonna happen! You have to start looking at weight loss realistically. There's a simple fat loss equation that is very simple yet very important – please take a note of this – 3500 calories equals one pound. That is just the truth. 3500 calories equals one pound.

However, people often have unrealistic goals, often thanks to Hollywood's false expectations. You see it happen on TV shows all the time: this person and that person lost 20 lbs in one week.

Is it possible to lose 20 lbs in one week? Absolutely. Is it possible to loose 20 lbs of *fat* in one week? Hell to the no!

For someone to loose 20 lbs of fat in one week, they would need to be in a 70,000 calorie deficit. That's impossible.

Consider this: Running on the treadmill for one hour burns an average of 500-700 calories. So, you'd have to spend 100-140 *hours* on the treadmill to lose 20 pounds. Given that there are only 168 hours in a week, how likely is that scenario?

The reason we assign reward and punishment to goals is because we, as humans, are emotional. We justify things with logic, but deep down, our decisions are purely emotional.

That's right, we're emotional. So it's much better if we accept that fact and learn to tie emotional reasons into our goals. My job at Fitness Concept is to figure out why people are looking to lose weight. I always ask clients, "Why are you here? Now, why are you *really* here? Why do you want to get in shape? Why did you show up today as opposed to last week?"

The reason I ask these questions is to find out their emotional "hot button" that I can use to light a fire under their A** and motivate them.

Here's an example. A lady came to me last year said, "I want to lose a few pounds." I asked, "Why today?" She responded, "I've been thinking about it for a while, and I just thought I would come in today."

"Yes, but why today, of all days? Why not last week or last month?" I pressed. After speaking to her and asking some very specific questions, I found out the emotional "hot button" of why she was at my gym that day.

The real reason that she was in my gym wanting to do personal training was that she was going to some kind of event in a couple of months. Her ex-husband was going to be there with his hot new wife, and she wanted to look just as good, if not better, to show her up.

Ladies and gentleman, that's an emotional reason. Do you think she got in shape? You bet!

That may seem like a silly reason to you, but the point is that it's an emotional reason, which we all have in some shape or another. For this woman, it was a specific event that she had to get ready for, and every time she came to the gym, and I would see her working out, I would just say, I saw the new wife and she's pretty hot. That simple statement had her working out harder and harder.

I want you to do the same. A good way to get motivation on your own is to buy a dress that you want to fit into and choose an event that you want to go to. Don't just window shop; actually buy the dress, even if it doesn't fit now. Tell yourself, "You know what, I don't fit quite right in that dress now but by Christmas time, I'm going to look really hot in that dress. I'm going to go to that Christmas party and everyone's going to go, 'Wow!'" Now, that's an emotional reason. Right?

So, here's what I want you to do, so you can start feeling great too. I want you to change your lifestyle. This is all about the long term. I don't want you to just go start an exercising and eating program and get good results right away, only to revert to your old ways and gain the weight back.

Remember, exercise and healthy eating should be like a marriage, not a casual relationship - and you don't want to end up divorced over one or two little slip-ups, do you?

As far as your health is concerned, you are either getting better or you are getting worse. There is no such thing as staying the same. So, set your goals continually. Your body is like a home improvement project. I don't know about you guys, but when I bought my home a long, long time ago, I mistakenly thought that I was done with spending money on it.

Are we ever really done improving our homes? The same goes with our bodies. The moment you are completely satisfied with the way you look is the moment you start regressing.

CHAPTER 1
The Proper Definition

Losing weight takes a lot of time, energy, and willpower if you want to get that perfect weight and figure you've always dreamed of. But before going through the **proper** step-by-step how-to's, let us first warm our minds up with the right information about this losing weight stuff. What's the real deal, anyway?

Health is Wealth

Being wealthy is neither about acquiring all the riches in the world nor getting whatever you want with just a snap of the fingers. It's more about investing something from an earlier period of your life and being able to continually use it until you grow old. No material thing can be such an investment because one day it comes, and before you know it, it's gone.

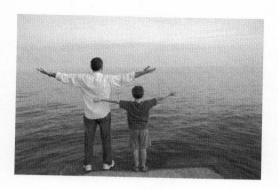

For instance, the money you earn today may be the car you'll be driving tomorrow. But automobiles don't last that long either; sooner or later, their parts will get rusty, until they become broken and useless in time. So much for the money you earned from hard work.

The real richness in this world is being happy in your life and satisfied with what you have – being able to do what you want to do, when you want to do it, and know that nothing will get in your way of accomplishing the things that will make you happy. However, if you're sick, these simple pleasures can be quickly taken from you. How can you play with a pet puppy if you can't stay close to it because you are allergic to its fur? How can you enjoy a pint of ice cream if you're not allowed to eat it because you're diabetic? Or, what good is a big house to live in when most of the time you stay in a hospital because of serious illnesses? In other words, money, riches, and other classy material things are no good at all when you can't be with them, eat them, or simply have them because certain sicknesses forbid you to, don't you agree?

What's better is not having any allergy to animal furs, even if you can't afford to buy a pet; not being diabetic, even if you don't have any ice cream for dessert; and staying in your own house even if it's not big enough to fit 3 people inside. When you are healthy and in perfect shape, the lack, or even absence, of material resources will not matter anymore. As long as you can do whatever you want to do, eat whatever your tongue feels like eating, and go wherever your feet bring you, you'll never be more content in your life - thus, making you wealthier than any rich-but-sick people out there.

Healthy People

People who are considered "healthy" are those who are physically and mentally fit. Physical fitness is the ability of the human body to function with vigor and alertness, without undue fatigue, and with ample energy to engage in leisure activities and meet physical stresses. Muscular strength, endurance, stamina, and general alertness are the overt signs of being physically fit.

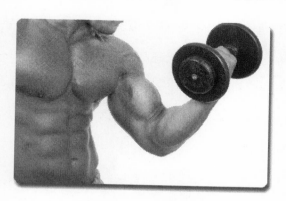

Your level of physical fitness can be influenced by regular, systematic exercise and proper nutrition. Moderate activity will maintain an individual at a level that is usually adequate to handle ordinary stress, while the right diet affects energy expenditure. Overweight, underweight, and weak individuals have low fitness levels.

On the other hand, mental fitness refers to a psychological state of well-being, characterized by continuing personal growth, a sense of purpose in life, self-acceptance, and positive relations with others.

Unhealthy People

In contrast with the above discussion, people who belong to the "unhealthy" category are the opposite of the healthy ones – unwell either in the body, the mind, or both. They are often physically ill or otherwise show symptoms of ill health, such as regular back pain. These sicknesses hinder them from performing daily activities properly, as you can see in the example below, where back pain is distracting this worker from his tasks.

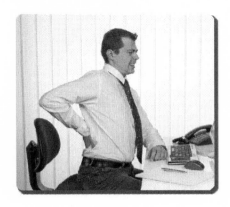

Unhealthy people get easily fatigued or stressed, resulting in unaccomplished tasks. The absence of exercise, or inappropriate exercise, and poor food intake is what makes people physically unfit.

Alternatively, people can also be mentally unhealthy if their psychological state is not well. Manifestations include always being doubtful, too much worrying, an inferiority complex, and negative relation to others.

Rate your Weight The Normal Way: Height-Weight Relationship

Physical health can be measured through the appropriateness of a person's weight to his height, where the body weight refers to the measure of one's heaviness and the height is the measure of his tallness.

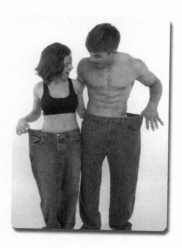

For instance, a woman measuring 5 ft high (1.52 m), with a medium body frame should weigh between 103 lbs to 115 lbs (46.72 kg – 52.16 kg) to be considered healthy. Another example: a man standing 5 ft 8 in (1.72 m) tall, with a large body frame, is healthy if he weighs between 144 lbs – 163 lbs (65.32 kg – 73.94 kg). Otherwise, if their weight is lower than the desired body weight for their height, they are considered underweight, and if, in turn, their weight is higher than the desired body weight for their height, they are said to be overweight. (See Appendix A for the chart of Desirable Weight Ranges.)

Body Mass Index (BMI)

Body Mass Index is a more accurate indicator of surplus body fat than kilos or pounds. It is a mathematical ratio of height to weight that can be linked with body composition (or body fat percentage) and with indices of health risk. Calculating BMI is as follows:

BMI = Weight (in kg) / Height (in m) x Height (in m)

or BMI = (Weight (in lbs) / Height (in inches) x Height (in inches)) x 700

For example, the calculation for someone weighing 80 kg (176 lbs) and 1.60 m (63 in) tall is:

BMI = $\frac{80 \text{ kg}}{(1.6 \times 16)}$ = 31.2

or BMI $= \frac{(176/(63 \times 63))}{} \times 700 = 31.0$

People with a BMI of 25.1 to 29.9 are considered overweight, and people with a BMI of 30 or above are considered obese. Thus, from the example above, a person weighing 80 kg and measuring 1.60 m tall is obese. A high BMI assumes a higher percentage of body fat, which places a person at a greater risk for developing chronic diseases and other serious illnesses.

BMI	Weight Category
Under 19	Underweight
20-25	Normal (Healthy)
25.1 – 29.9	Overweight
30 & above	Obese

Table 1.1 Body weight categories according to BMI

However, for some people, the BMI is not a reliable indication of health. A highly-muscled individual who is very fit and healthy may have a somewhat heavy body weight because muscles pack on a lot of pounds. This person may have a high BMI that improperly puts him or her in the overweight or obese categories. Likewise, thin individuals who have a low body weight with very little muscle and a higher percentage of fat may have a normal BMI, which would be an incorrect indication of healthiness.

No Affinity for Obesity

Obesity is defined as being 20 percent or more above one's desirable weight range (see appendix A again for reference). It is a medical condition that refers mainly to storage of excess body fat. The human body naturally stores fat tissue under the skin and around organs and joints. Fat is critical for good health because it is a source of energy when the body lacks the natural energy necessary to sustain life processes, and it provides insulation and protection for internal organs. But the accumulation of too much fat in the body is associated with a variety of health problems.

Causes of Excess Weight Gain

A calorie is the unit used to measure the energy value of food and the energy used by the body to maintain normal functions. When the calories from food intake equal the calories of energy the body uses, weight remains constant. But when more calories are eaten than the body needs, the body stores those additional calories as fat, causing subsequent weight gain. One pound (1 lb) of fat represents about 3,500 excess calories.

Obesity is partially determined by a person's genetic makeup. If a child inherited the excessive body fat cells of his obese parents, more likely, he will tend to eat more than his body needs; thus, making him obese too. Copying the poor eating habits of parents also affects a child's body weight.

Lifestyles also play a key role in the triggering of obesity. Eating big servings of food at restaurants and fast food joints more frequently than nutritious, home-cooked foods could add more calories and fats to your diet. Also, devoting little to no time to exercise and other physical activities does not control weight gain either. You can also promote an inactive lifestyle by filling your time with non-physical recreational activities such as browsing the internet, playing video games, watching movies, and lounging in front of the television, along with using laborsaving devices of the modern living, such as personal computers, telephones, and remote controls

Effects and Possible Complications of Excess Weight

Obesity increases the risk of developing disease. Possible complications include:

- Heart disease

- High blood pressure

- Cancer

- Diabetes

- Gallbladder disease

- Breathing problems

- Bloating and stomach upsets

- Varicose veins

- Severe psychological problems

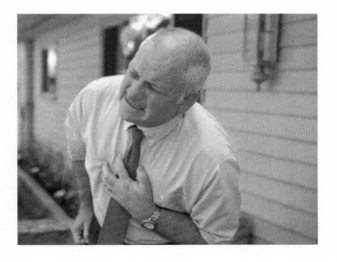

In fact, according to some studies, almost 70 percent of heart disease cases in the United States are linked to excess body fat, and obese people are more than twice as likely to develop high blood pressure as their thinner counterparts. Obese women are at nearly twice the risk for developing breast cancer, and all obese people have an estimated 42 percent higher chance of developing colon cancer. Almost 80 percent of patients with Type 2, or non-insulin-dependent, diabetes mellitus are obese. The risk of medical complications, particularly heart disease, increases when body fat is distributed around the waist, especially in the abdomen. This type of upper body fat distribution is more common in men than in women.

The social and psychological problems experienced by obese people are also challenging. Discrimination of "fat" people is most likely to occur in educational institutions, employment, and social relationships. Other psychological effects include stress, nervous tension, boredom, frustration, lack of friends, depression, inferiority complex, and poor self-esteem.

CHAPTER 2
The Proper Plan

Before taking action in any problem we encounter, there should always be a plan first (that is, if we want to come up with positive results). You wouldn't want to enter a battle without preparing how to defeat the enemy, would you? Operating a task without planning is like building a house without a blueprint or playing basketball without a team play with your teammates. How would you expect a good outcome?

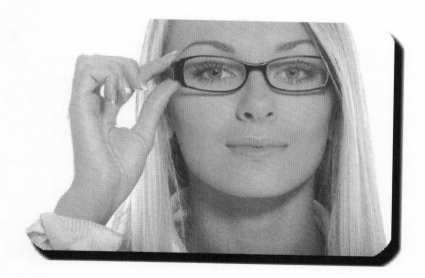

Losing weight is not at all different from the above mentioned plan-necessity situations. It also involves taking the right actions and finding the proper ways that need to be perfectly planned in order to bring satisfying results.

Setting a Goal

Okay, so let's say your weight is 20% above what's considered normal for your height. You tend to eat more than 5 regular meals each day. You're certain that you're physically unfit. Now, the question is: what do you want to happen?

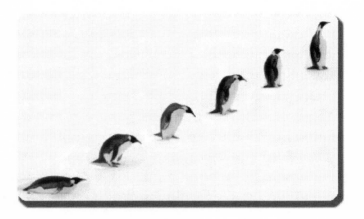

Setting a goal is the first step in planning. Know what you want to accomplish. This way, the road you are taking is clear. You can keep track of your journey – and find out whether or not you are going along the right direction. With a goal in mind, you will find yourself more motivated to finish a task, or, in some cases, to start one.

Be Definite

Setting a specific goal, when planning to lose weight, improves your chances of success. Be clear and definite with what you want to happen. Vague aims such as "I'd like to be healthier," or "I need to lose a few kilos," tend to produce half-hearted efforts and poor results. Instead, state your goal distinctly: "I want to lose 2-3 kilos this week and every week for two months," or "I will trim my waistline from 40 inches down to 32 inches by the end of the month." If you need to, write your goal down and put it where you will always be able to see - and read - it. This way, you'll always be reminded of what you want and need to accomplish by the end of the month, the week, or even the day.

Be Realistic

In establishing a definite goal, make sure that it is possible and doable – or realistic, in simpler terms. How can a goal like "I'll lose 15 lbs in just a week" happen if even the most reasonable weight-loss diet suggests that you can only burn 6-7 lbs in a week? And that is if you follow strictly what the diet recommends, with no cheating.

Goals need to be sensible so that they won't be far from coming true. What happens when you set a goal that you can't possibly achieve, no matter how hard you try, is that you will only get depressed and disappointed, which are some of the psychological causes of obesity. And the problem just goes in circles without an end in sight.

Be Strategic

After carefully deliberating a goal of what you want to achieve, the next step is planning how to accomplish it. Planning involves proper scheduling of activities, including exercises, meals, and sleeping and waking, to be done throughout the whole day for a certain period of time. This schedule should be comprised of the time these activities should be done, the duration they will take, and, in the case of eating meals, the food to be consumed. This way, inappropriate, spur-of-the-moments decisions can be avoided because your day will already be planned out.

A proper and effective plan should give you enough time to perform such activities. That is, ample time should be given to be able to meet the objectives correctly. For example, sleep should be scheduled to last for around 7 to 8 hours a day so that you'll be able to get enough rest. Lack of sleep may cause improper eating habits the next day.

Again, plans should be relatively realistic. Include only time and activities you know that you can accomplish in a given period of time. Also, as you finish preparing the plan, you might want to write it down since you can't always keep all of the details in mind. Post your plan in a place where you can always see it so that it will often remind you what your plans are for the day. Try your best not to skip anything in your scheduled plan so as not to ruin the effectiveness of the overall plan.

On the following pages, you'll find an example of an effective scheduled plan.

DAY 1

Around 7 hours of sleep

1 hour of exercise after waking up: breathing exercises and jogging

Breakfast: High Fiber Cereal with non fat milk.

Lunch: 1 cup brown rice, vegetables, grilled chicken water

Snack: Apple and cottage cheese

Dinner: Mixed green salad with tuna and low fat dressing.

10-minute breathing exercise before going to bed

DAY 2

Around 7 hours of sleep

1 hour exercise after waking up: breathing exercises and jump rope

Breakfast: Whole wheat toast, sliced tomatoes, cottage cheese.

Lunch: Turkey breast, red potatoes, spinach.

Snack: Sliced Mangos

Dinner: Chicken breast, asparagus. chicken soup, banana,

ChChickewater

10-minute breathing exercise and crunches before going to bed

AM

6:00	Wake up
6:00-7:00	Exercise: Breathing & jogging
7:00-8:00	Prepare & eat breakfast: (Egg whites, oatmeal)

PM

12:00-1:00	Prepare & eat lunch: (Brown rice, veggies, water, Chicken breast)
3:30-4:00	Snacks (Apple and cottage cheese
6:30-7:30	Prepare & eat dinner: (Mixed green salad, tuna, low fat dressing.
10:00-10:10	Breathing exercise
11:00	Bedtime

AM

6:00	Wake up
6:00-7:00	Exercise: Breathing & jumping rope
7:00-8:00	Prepare & eat breakfast: (Whole wheat toast, cottage cheese, sliced tomatoes.)

PM

12:00-1:00	Prepare and eat lunch: (Turkey breast, spinach, red potato)
3:30-4:00	Snacks Mango slices
6:30-7:30	Prepare & eat dinner: (Chicken breast, asparagus
10:00	Exercise: Breathing & 10 Crunches
11:00	Bedtime

A sound plan for someone to lose weight looks like this:

Plan according to the examples above. Remember that adequate sleep, regular exercise, and healthy meals are the most essential elements to include in your daily schedule. Take note of your calorie intake (through foods) and calorie burning (through exercising) for efficient results. (See Appendix B for Food Calories and compare it with Appendix C for Calorie-Burning Exercises.)

The Role of Positive Thinking

The earlier-mentioned goals can be re-stated as affirmations, such as "I will lose 3 lbs this week," or "I will trim my waistline down 10 inches." Affirmations are positive thoughts that, when truly believed, will somehow help to make things happen. Positive thinking produces positive reality by triggering our body to do what it says, thus, providing you with willpower. For example, if you truly believe that you will lose 3 lbs this week, your thoughts will command your body to do specific things this week in order to lose those 3 lbs - until your goal becomes a reality.

Affirmations, or positive statements about yourself or your intentions, are a deceptively simple aid to achieving a goal.

They work by imprinting themselves upon the subconscious mind through regular repetition – saying, reading, or writing them down over and over again. Some people even record their affirmations on audio tapes and listen to them repeatedly to make sure that the thoughts are planted on their mind.

If you truly mean your affirmations and want them to come true, then they will. This practice does require a little discipline, but the benefits will surely outweigh the time and effort you spend.

CHAPTER 3
Why You Should Never Go Hungry

Now, every one of us has gone through what we call a starvation diet, where we starve ourselves to lose weight. For some reason, we associate starving with fat loss and weight loss. That's not true.

This is very important and is the basis of why so many people fail. Remember, the moment you are hungry, you are doing something wrong. You should never go hungry. You should never *be* hungry. Here's why: when you are hungry, you tend to overeat. This is so important, I'm going to repeat that: Not eating leads to overeating. When you are hungry, there's a strong temptation to sit down and eat everything in site. To avoid this, don't skip meals!

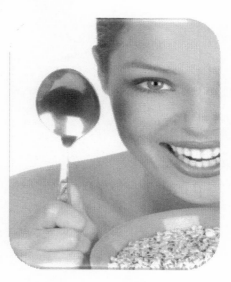

Besides, a diet that's too low in calories makes you lose muscle. Why is that important? When we miss meals and go hungry, we go catabolic. When our bodies go catabolic, we not only lose body fat, but we lose muscle as well. Muscle is a metabolically-active tissue, which means that the less muscle you have, the less metabolism you have – and because a higher metabolism helps you burn fat quicker and easier, less muscle is going to make fat loss that much harder.

More muscle mass – and therefore a higher metabolism – is one reason why men lose fat faster than women.

Having more muscle is like having a bigger engine. A big V8 engine burns a lot more fuel than a smaller 4-cylinder engine.

If you go on a very low calorie diet, you will be hungry. I don't know about you, but I am one of the most pig-headed, self-disciplined guys out there. My wife will definitely agree to that. If I'm starving and there is junk food in front of me, guess what? I want to eat it. So, you never want to put yourself in that position. That is why you should never, ever, ever, ever go hungry. Don't worry; we will show you how you can do that.

Also, your brain works on glucose. So, on a very low-calorie diet, you will find yourself confused and unable to concentrate and work. Trust me when I tell you that I have failed a physics test in college, even when I knew all the material…all because I wasn't taking in enough calories.

I have run a red light because I was zoning out, again thanks to calorie deficiency. Trust me – you don't want to find yourself in that situation! I have been there, done that, and now I am here to teach you how to get results the fastest, safest way possible.

Starvation diets decrease your thyroid output

Hey, listen, our bodies are the most efficient things ever. Our bodies are designed to do one thing and one thing only, and that's survive. Your body doesn't know that you are trying to lose weight. Our bodies are governed by what is called a negative feedback system. What do I mean by that? Remember that your body is meant to do one thing and one thing only. Write this down, this is very important. Your body is made to survive. Your body does not know that all of a sudden you are starving yourself because you want to lose body fat. Even though we are in the year 2010, your body was designed 10,000 years ago. So your genetics are still 10,000 years behind. So when you start starving yourself, your body thinks, "Oh my god, we are not getting any food!" You are not catching a tiger. You are not catching any lions. So, you are not going to get any food. Therefore, in order to survive during times of starvation, tour bodies slow down the thyroid output, in true survival mode.

When your thyroid output decreases, so does your body temperature. That's how you can tell when somebody is on a really crazy diet. They are cold all the time.

When your thyroid hormone decreases, your body temperature decreases and then your metabolism decreases. That is what we don't want. Without getting into medical terms, what happens is the conversion of thyroxin, which is normally T4, to the more potent T3 triiodine; this decrease happens through an enzymatic process.

Also, remember that because of the starvation diet, you lose fat weight, then you lose muscle, and then one day you drop the diet and eat normal. You gain the weight back, plus you gain even more weight now because you lost muscle, which, you might remember, leads to a decreased metabolism.

Oprah Winfrey comes to mind when I think of this scenario.

I never know which Oprah's going to show up onscreen. Is it going to be the big Oprah? Is it going to be the skinny Oprah? Why does this happen? Because Oprah, even with all her money and all her trainers, still hasn't changed her lifestyle. You have got to change your lifestyle if you want permanent results.

Weight vs Body Composition

So, let's talk about weight. Weight is pretty meaningless, actually. The body composition is what is more important. When you weigh in, your trainers are just making sure you are heading in the right direction. Otherwise, weight doesn't mean much. Let me give you an example. I'm about 5'5" and I weigh 185lb. My wife still thinks I'm 5'7" (that's a whole another story - I told her that when we started dating since she is 5'9").

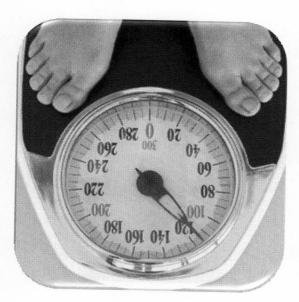

Body fat percentage is the measure of your body composition. It tells what your body is made out of. Remember,

80% of your body is water, so you will see fluctuations in your weight. Don't drive yourself crazy with these little fluctuations in your weight.

By the way, I recommend weighing yourself once a week at the same time each day and with the same scale. You will always gain a few pounds by each evening due to water you've drank and food you've eaten throughout the day, so if you weigh yourself at night one day and in the morning another, you won't get accurate results.

Okay, let's talk about ideal body fat percentage. For men, normal is 12-18%, and for women, it is 18-24%. Men with a body fat percentage over 35% are considered obese, while women whose percentage is over 40% are considered obese.

Your body and your checking account are very similar

Let's talk about calories, because I've found that people usually want to talk about calories this and calories that. What it comes down to is this: Your body is like your bank account. What happens when you deposit more in your bank account than you take out? The balance is going to get bigger, right? That's not happening to too many of us these days, but that's what happens. If you take out more from the bank than you put in, your bank account is going to get smaller. Likewise, if you burn more calories than you eat, your body will get smaller too. The bottom line is that if you deposit more than you take out, you'll gain more. It is that simple. So, then, your body will just store the extra amounts as body fat if you eat too much, right? I don't necessarily agree with that idea. Is it really true? Yeah, hypothetically it is true. Hypothetically, you can eat too much broccoli and asparagus, chicken, fish, and oatmeal, I guess. Is that really possible?

Let's look at an example:

As a rule of thumb, if you want to:

Lose weight: your weight x 10 = daily calories needed

Maintain weight: your weight x 12 = daily calories needed

Gain weight: your weight x 15 = daily calories needed

So, let's say that my client weighs 200 lbs. He/she must consume 2,000 or less calories per day to lose weight.

Ladies and gentleman, it is extremely hard NOT to lose weight if you're eating foods that:

1) Are Nutritious

2) Are Filling

3) Don't have many calories

Make sure to see the resource section of this book to find these kind of foods.

I got down to 2.7% body fat and easily won bodybuilding title after bodybuilding title by using the same methods that I am teaching you here.

So, back to the example above, my client is 200 lbs and wants to lose weight.

Let's just say that he has a healthy appetite, and he eats the following today:

Breakfast

8 egg whites

½ cup oatmeal

Sliced tomatoes

Total Calories: 350

Snack

A can of tuna in water

An apple

Total Calories: 250

Lunch

4 oz chicken breast

½ cup of brown rice

1 cup of broccoli

Total Calories: 300

Snack

35 grams of whey protein

Total Calories: 150

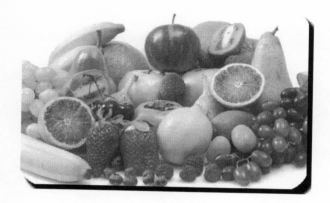

Dinner

4-5 oz halibut

2 small red potatoes

5 asparagus

Total Calories: 250

Snack

½ cup of 2% cottage cheese

Total Calories: 100

So, the grand total of calories for the day would be 1,400 calories, which is way below the 2,000 calories needed for weight loss.

The above example explains why most of my clients tell me that they seem to eat all day long and still manage to lose weight.

After all, who cares about losing weight if you are constantly starving and walking around miserable?

With so much misinformation out there today, so many people are confused and end up making weight loss more complicated then it really is.

Remember, if your weight loss plan is too complicated, you are not going to stick with it. Always ask yourself one question whenever you approach any exercise and nutrition program: Can I do this for the rest of my life?

If the answer is no, then don't do even bother starting. Remember, for this to work, it must be a lifestyle change. It's no wonder you see people yo-yo up and down with their weight for years; they never change their LIFESTYLE.

A lot of people sweat the little things, and they're like, "Oh my gosh, how much chicken breast should I eat, how many egg whites should I eat, how much broccoli?" Then they worry so much that they don't eat enough and end up crashing and devouring a chocolate cake later. I want you to eat good food all day long, as long as you are eating good food from that A and A+ list in the resource section in the back of this book, and you won't run into this problem.

I have never seen anyone gain weight by eating too much brown rice, chicken breast and oatmeal.

The problem with our society, and why we tend to crash at night, is because we are living in a busy society where we are going, going, going all the time. We tend to eat out of convenience.

We always seem to be in a hurry. Following is a typical scenario that I see in my facility all the time:

We wake up in the morning and rush to get ready to go to work, take the kids to school, etc., so we tend to skip breakfast (a very bad idea, especially since you haven't eaten in 6-12 hours) or have a quick convenient grab-and-go breakfast (usually coffee with a sugary snack).

Then we go to work, rush into deadlines, and get caught up with everything at work, usually skipping the mid-morning snack or having "junk" food that people bring into offices.

Lunch usually consists of fast food or other processed foods that we can grab and go. We come back to the office and work, work and more work.

We come home starving after a day of not eating and, thanks to malnutrition, eat everything in site. Then we sit on the couch, watching the tube, and go to bed.

You see, sooner or later you have to catch up with your calorie requirement. It's much better to eat small, frequent, nutritious meals than to crash and have one huge meal at the time when you are least active (night time).

Why dieticians are dead wrong in their approach

I remember when, a few years ago, I hired a dietician to come into our facility and do nutrition consults with my clients.

I soon had to come back and take over as our clients were nor seeing results.

Here is something that dieticians will tell you: Small amounts of anything, even junk food, will probably not get stored as body fat if you are eating less than you are supposed to eat, basically saying that a calorie is a calorie. Is this true or not true? Technically, it is supposed to be true, right? But I want you guys to always, always question when somebody tells you something. Don't take my word for it, and don't take anybody else's word for it. Is a calorie a calorie? There are dieticians out there that tell you as long as you stay within this many points or this many calories, you are good. So, for example, let's say I got up this morning and wanted to have a cake. If the cake has all the calories that I need for that day, then that means I am OK as long as 1 don't as I don't eat anything else that day. Sound right to you?

So the question is: Are all calories equal? Consider if we all had a identical twin who ate 2,000 calories per day from nothing but low-fat protein sources, low-glycemic starches, green veggies and fruits.

You, on the other hand, choose to eat 2,000 calories from fried foods and sugary snacks.

Would you and your twin look the same after a year, providing that the physical activity remained the same for both of you?

Of course not!!!

So, calories are not all created equal.

A calorie is not just a calorie; it is the quality of the food that counts. There are a lot of more things involved than just the amount of calories you eat. What I'm trying to tell you is this: don't try to count calories all the time, because you are going to drive yourself crazy. You are not going to weigh and measure food for the rest of your life. You just aren't going to be able to do that. Even in the height of my career as a body builder, I didn't do that. So, all I want you to do is focus on eating small, frequent meals with the right amount of macro nutrients. I'm going to talk about that right here, right now.

This is going to be the key difference between those of you who are going to get results and those of you who won't. This is the key! Are you ready? Write this down. This is the different between my clients that come to my gym and see weight loss and clients who come to the gym and see mediocre results.

The most important factor in fat loss

Meal frequency alone has a miraculous effect on human physiology.

You get to eat five, or even six, small meals a day. As soon as you get up, you have to start your engine with a good breakfast and then, every two and a half or three hours after that, you have to eat again to keep your blood sugar level steady. That is the key: keeping your blood sugar level steady.

Skipping a meal is the cardinal sin of fat burning. People tell me, "Sam, I only eat one time per day, so I don't know why I'm gaining so much weight." It's because in that one time, you were so hungry that you ate 3,000 calories. At any given time, if you give your body too much food, your body is not going to be able to metabolize all of it; therefore, it's going to store the extra as body fat.

Benefits of Eating Small, Frequent Meals

1) Eating small, frequent meals speeds up your metabolism by a process known as thermic effect of food.

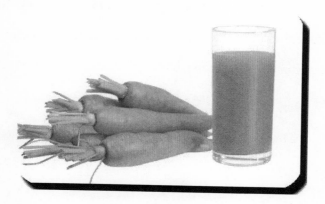

Thermic effect of food (also commonly known simply as thermic effect when the context is known), or TEF in shorthand, is the increment in energy expenditure above resting metabolic rate due to the cost of processing food for storage and use. It is one of the components of metabolism, along with the resting metabolic rate and the exercise component. Another term commonly used to describe this component of total metabolism is the specific dynamic action (SDA). A common number used to estimate the magnitude of the thermic effect of food is about 10% of the caloric intake of a given time period, though the effect varies substantially for different food components. Dietary fat is very easy to process and has very little thermic effect, while protein is hard to process and has a much larger thermic effect.

Raw celery and grapefruit are often claimed to have negative caloric balance (which means that they take more energy to digest than usable energy received from the food), presumably because the thermic effect is greater than the caloric content due to the high fibre matrix that must be unraveled to access their carbohydrates; there has been no research carried out to test this theory, however.

The thermic effect of food is increased by both aerobic training of sufficient duration and intensity and by anaerobic weight training. However, the increase is marginal, amounting to 7-8 calories per hour. The primary determinants of daily TEF are the quantity and composition of the food ingested.

Skipping meals may seem like the quickest way to lose weight, but it could do more harm than good. Think of your metabolism as a fat-burning machine; if you don't give it the fuel it needs, it'll stop working. And that's just what happens when you skip meals, especially breakfast. Eating breakfast in the morning jump-starts your metabolism. Then, eating several small meals during the day keeps it running. Skipping meals causes your body to go into fasting mode and slows down your metabolism, while causing your body to hold onto the fat it has stored. Plus, research shows that skipping one meal can cause you to overeat at the next. So, not only are you slowing your metabolism, you're actually eating more calories. No wonder you're not losing weight!

I view skipping meals as being similar to hibernation for animals. Hibernation allows animals to conserve energy during the winter when food is in short supply. During hibernation, animals drastically lower their metabolism so as to tap energy reserves stored as body fat at a slower rate than if they were awake and active.

2. Frequent meals prevent binges and control cravings.

Skipping a meal causes the blood sugar levels to drop, which leads to overeating at the next meal or eating later in the evening, when the body's ability to burn and utilize calories efficiently slows down and the body begins to naturally hold onto calories. For this reason, I recommend eating four to six smaller meals throughout the day.

3. Frequent meals help maintain high energy levels by regulating blood sugar and insulin levels.

When you eat carbohydrates, they're digested and absorbed into the bloodstream in the form of glucose (blood sugar). This triggers the pancreas to release the hormone known as insulin. The amount of insulin released will correspond to the amount and type of carbohydrates consumed. When small amounts of carbohydrates and insulin-stimulating foods are consumed, there's a small output of insulin. When large amounts of carbohydrates and insulin-stimulating foods are consumed, there is a large rise in insulin.

When carbohydrates are consumed alone, there's a faster rise in insulin than when they're consumed in combination with protein. When simple, refined carbohydrates are consumed, there's also a greater rise in insulin. One of insulin's jobs is to transport the glucose from the bloodstream into the cells, where it can be used for energy or stored as glycogen for later use.

Avoid Feeling Hungry While Losing Weight

Here are a few tips to help you avoid hunger during your weight-loss efforts:

- Drink a lot of water.

- Eat small, frequent meals to fire up your metabolism and **stop feeling hungry**.

- Eat plenty of protein to feel full.

- Fill up on fiber. High-fiber foods add bulk to your diet, making you **feel satisfied longer**.

- Eat slowly to give your brain a chance to signal that you are full.

- Don't over-exercise, as it will cause you to be hungrier and – therefore – eat more.

- Wait 20 minutes before giving in to food cravings.

- Create a list of hobbies or activities to do in place of eating.

- Don't ignore your body's hunger signals. Eat a light meal of a nutritious snack at the first sign of hunger.

- Avoid fad diets that promise overnight weight-loss results.

- Manage stress without turning to food.

- Get plenty of sleep. Being well rested will allows you to fight off hunger pains and low energy levels.

The ultimate meal combination

Below you will see the "Top 10 Lists" of what I eat every day or almost every day. Exact quantities and menus are not listed, just the foods.

Of course, my food intake varies. I aim to get as many different varieties of fruits and vegetables as possible over the course of every week and there are a lot of substitutions made, so you are not seeing my full list here. This is just what I eat the most of every day.

I also want to point out that while I don't believe that an extremely low-carb diet is necessary or most effective when you look at the long term, I do reduce my carb intake moderately and temporarily prior to body building competitions, so my starchy carb and grain intake goes down during that brief pre-competition period when I'm working on that really "ripped" look (I do eat lots and lots of veggies, though!).

This list reflects my personal preferences, so this is not a prescription for all readers to eat as I do.

It's very important for long-term compliance to choose foods YOU enjoy and to have the option for a wide variety of choices. In the past several years, nutrition and obesity research - looking at ALL types of diets - has continued to end with the conclusion that almost any diet that is not completely moronic can work in the short term.

It's not so much about the high carb, low carb argument or any other debate as much as it is about compliance, or sticking to the diet. The trouble is, restricted diets and staying in a calorie deficit is HARD in general, so because most people can't stick with any program, they fall off the wagon, whichever wagon that may be.

I believe that a lot of our attention needs to shift away from pointless debates (low carb vs. high carb is getting really old…like…get over it everyone, it's <u>a calorie deficit</u> that makes you lose weight, not the amount of carbs, whether they're high or low).

Instead, our focus should shift towards building an eating program that we can enjoy more while still getting us leaner and healthier, and especially towards **building an eating program that improves compliance** (and that includes using <u>emotional</u>

and psychological techniques that can improve compliance as well).

Here's one good answer: Eat foods you ENJOY that still fit within healthy, fat-burning, muscle-building guidelines!

On the next page are the foods I choose to achieve this outcome. This eating plan is not difficult to stick with at all, by the way. I enjoy eating like this and it feels almost weird NOT to eat like this after doing it for so long. Remember, habits work in both directions, and as Jim Rohn said, *"Bad habits are easy to form and hard to live with and good habits are hard to form but easy to live with."*

The following foods are listed in the order I frequently consume them. So, for example, if oatmeal is on the top of the list, that means this is the food I am most likely to eat every single day.

My 10 top starchy carb and grains

1. Oatmeal (old fashioned)

2. Yams (almost the same as sweet potatoes)

3. brown rice (I love basmati, a long-grain aromatic rice)

4. Sweet potatoes

5. Multi-grain hot cereal (mix or barley, oats, rye triticale and a few others)

6. White potatoes (glycemic index be damned!)

7. 100% whole wheat bread

8. 100% whole wheat pasta

9. Beans (great for healthy chili recipes)

10. Cream of rice hot cereal

My Top 10 top vegetables

1. Broccoli

2. Asparagus

3. Spinach

4. Salad greens

5. Tomatoes

6. Peppers (green and red)

7. Onions

8. Mushrooms

9. Cucumbers

10. Zucchini

My top 10 lean proteins

1. Egg whites

2. Whey protein (protein powder supplement)

3. Chicken breast

4. Salmon (wild Alaskan)

5. Turkey breast

6. Top round steak (grass-fed beef)

7. Flank steak (grass-fed beef)

8. Cod fish

9. Bison/Buffalo

10. Rainbow Trout

My top 10 fruits

1. Grapefruit

2. Apples

3. Blueberries

4. Cantaloupe

5. Oranges

6. Bananas

7. Peaches

8. Grapes

9. Strawberries

10. Pineapple

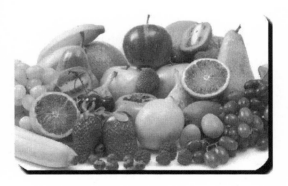

By the way, remember - fruit is nature's candy!

And also note that I DO include healthy fats as well, such as walnuts, almonds, olive oil, flaxseeds, flaxseed oil (supplement

- not to cook with), avocado and a few others that are slipping my mind at the moment.

Also, YES I eat dairy and I have nothing against it, nor am I lactose intolerant. I just don' t eat as much dairy as the rest of the stuff on my lists. When I eat dairy, its usually skim milk, low- or non-fat cottage cheese, low- or non-fat yogurt, and low- or non-fat cheese (I love cheese and egg white omelettes).

Hope you found this list helpful and interesting. Keep in mind that this is MY food list, and although you probably couldn't go wrong to emulate it, you need to choose foods you enjoy in order to develop habits you can stick with long term. There are, for example, hundreds of other fruits and vegetables out there...enjoy them all!

Top 5 Ways to Lose Fat and Keep Muscle

Don't Starve Yourself

Not even the most sleek sports car can function without fuel. Many people aiming for fat-loss and weight-loss goals attempt to lower their caloric intake drastically to get quick results.

While a drastic reduction in calories will cause you to lose weight, the most at the outset will be due to water weight, and it is not a long-term solution.

People who use starvation to lose weight gain it back almost 100% of the time.

Proper weight loss is all about elevating the metabolism with exercise while maintaining a healthy, balanced diet and lifestyle that can be maintained over the course of a lifetime.

Obtain a sufficient amount of protein in your diet

Your muscles are made up of protein, so obviously you need to consume protein to maintain your muscle during fat-loss goals.

This is not to say that carbohydrates and essential fats are less important, but protein is what makes up your muscles.

Protein causes you to feel satisfied after you consume meals with a significant portion of protein. Dietary protein also costs your body more energy to break down, burning some extra calories in the process.

A common belief is that protein builds muscles, which is not entirely the case. With proper training as a stimulus, dietary protein can help you build muscle, but it doesn't do the work on its own.

During fat-loss diets, protein plays an important role in the maintenance of your lean body mass (muscle), which contributes to your metabolism.

If you make a plan to lower your caloric intake and perform intense exercise, obtaining enough protein in your diet through lean meats, dairy products, vegetable sources and protein supplements can help you keep your muscle while your elevated metabolism does the job to get rid of fat.

Keep Exercise Sessions Short and Sweet

Spend less time working out by exercising smart.

Intensity and duration have an inverse relationship. In other words, the longer you work out, the less intense your workout is.

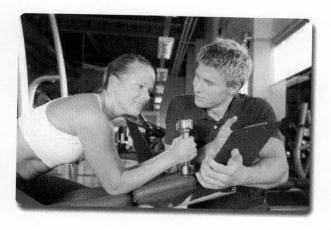

Think about this the next time you are in the gym for two hours. Fat loss is all about keeping your metabolism elevated so your body is constantly burning calories around the clock.

Short, high-intensity exercise sessions have a high after-burn. You will burn calories at an accelerated rate during the recovery process if you perform a short-duration workout.

During short-duration, high-intensity workouts, you are also highly unlikely to catabolize (break down) your own muscle as opposed to longer duration workouts, provided you are not starving yourself.

Since high-intensity workouts take more time to recover from, you may want to mix in some longer duration, lower intensity workouts. Listen to your body, and you will achieve your fat-loss goals most efficiently.

Have a proper post-workout recovery You have a 30 minute "window of opportunity" after every workout.

Many gym-goers and even clients of personal trainers make the huge mistake of not "refueling" **properly** after weight training and cardiovascular workouts.

After you work out, your body is starving for nutrients, specifically carbohydrates. In order to jump-start your recovery and progress towards achieving your goals, you must intake a good amount of carbohydrates and a little bit of protein directly after your workouts.

Many people also make the mistake of only taking protein supplements after training, which is also a big mistake.

Carbohydrates not only spare the body a loss of proteins after a workout but also help create the blood sugar and insulin response that shuttles the protein to the micro-damaged muscles to begin the reparation process.

The misconception exists that you burn fat during and after your workouts. A proper, easily digestible carbohydrate and protein mixture (in liquid form) is very important to take directly following weight training and cardio workouts, regardless of whether your fitness goals include fat loss, weight loss, toning, or strength training.

Perform Weight training

The primary function of weight training is NOT building muscle!

Maintaining lean body mass is the primary function of weight training. Even if your primary goal is to lose a large amount of weight, weight training is a great way to keep your fat-burning metabolism high while you lose weight.

Many people fear that weight training makes it more difficult to lose weight and burn fat, but this belief could not be further from the truth.

Whether you gain or lose weight from weight training is entirely dependent upon your diet. If you are on a fat-loss program with a workout mixture of weight training and cardio and a low-calorie, balanced diet, the combination will help you lose weight and burn fat.

It is very difficult for men and virtually impossible for women to gain "too much muscle" from weight training. A proper weight-training program, including exercises for all of the major muscle groups through different movement planes and ranges of motion, will do wonders for the human body and especially for fat loss.

Understanding macronutrients

Macronutrients are carbohydrates, proteins and fats. Let's start with carbohydrates. Carbohydrates are your muscle's primary energy source. During exercise, your muscles need a continuous supply of energy from carbohydrates, proteins and fats that are in the muscle, liver and bloodstream. The intensity and duration of activity determine their predominance of which macronutrient is burned. But carbohydrates are the primary source of energy for muscles, as well as all of your body's main tissues. Almost all dietary carbohydrates come from plant sources, with the exception of lactose, which is found in milk.

Carbohydrates are made up of carbon, hydrogen, and oxygen and created through a process in plants that absorbs energy from the sun and converts it into carbohydrates that the plant uses for energy and stores within itself. When we eat these plants, we, in turn, are eating carbohydrates. Carbohydrates are the only source of energy that the brain and central nervous system use. It is thought that the brain and central nervous system need about 130 grams of glucose a day. Our muscles also need a steady supply of carbohydrates in the basic form of glucose to contract and move.

Carbohydrates also have spare muscle protein from being used to create energy and metabolize fat efficiently. Some carbohydrate is needed in every diet. Carbohydrate ratios supply beneficial fiber to your diet that neither protein nor fat provide. The minimum amount of carbohydrates needed daily to prevent a deficiency is the recommended dietary amount of 130 grams of carbohydrates within an intake of 20 to 35 grams of fiber per day.

Types of Carbohydrates

Carbohydrates are classified, or named, by their chemical structure. Monosaccharides are single-unit carbohydrates, diasaccharides are two monosaccharides linked together, and polysaccharides are carbohydrates with multiple single-unit sugar molecules linked together to form one long chain of carbohydrates. Generally, most experts refer to carbohydrates as either simple, meaning one- or two-unit molecules, or complex for the long-chain polymers. Although there are some exceptions to the rule, simple carbohydrates are usually sugars or sweeteners, and complex carbohydrates are starches or fibers. A healthful diet would obtain the majority of these carbohydrates from fruits, vegetables, whole grains, vegetables, cereals, and lean dairy products. Limiting added sugars and sweeteners is being recommended by several health organizations in an effort to curb obesity in the United States.

Carbohydrates are the major source of energy during exercise and low–intensity movements; with workouts that require less than 60% of your VO2 max fat oxidation can supply enough energy for exercise. 1. Fatty acids can supply the majority of energy while exercising at a lower intensity for several hours. As the intensity picks up, however, so does the reliance on carbohydrates to fuel muscles. . For example, if you are doing an all-out 100m sprint, carbohydrates will supply 100% of the energy. As carbohydrates run low in the body, you have to slow down. Muscles have a limited supply of glycogen, the storage form of carbohydrates. A typical person will have 300 grams to 400 grams or 1200 to 1600 calories worth of carbohydrates stored in their muscles. Of those, 300 to 400 calories are usually stored in the liver and 100 calories in the bloodstream. The body can store a maximum of just over 2,000 calories worth of carbohydrates to be burned during exercise.

Studies have shown that eating a high carbohydrate diet ensures that your body has adequate muscle and liver stores of carbohydrates to burn. Because your body only has a limited supply of stored carbohydrates, it is important to consume additional carbohydrates during high-intensity events if you want to be able to exercise at a higher intensity. The harder and longer you exercise, the more carbohydrates your muscles need to store. Without adequate carbohydrates in your diet, you may experience tiredness and lack of motivation to train. Carbohydrates are essential for mental acuity as well. So if you need to be sharp in your particular sport, don't skimp on carbohydrates. In addition, consuming carbohydrates during those activities helps reduce fatigue and also helps us perceive the exercise as being easier.

Chronic training or lack of carbohydrates have been linked to symptoms of over-training and may even compromise your immune system. Not all carbohydrates are created equal, however; let's take a look at them in more detail now.

Understanding Glycemic Index and Glycemic Load

Glycemic index is a term that everyone is talking about these days but that is greatly misunderstood. The glycemic index is a measurement to rank how fast a carbohydrate is digested and absorbed, resulting in a rise in blood sugar level. It's a way to compare foods gram for gram based on their effects on blood glucose levels. Carbohydrates that break down quickly have the highest glycemic indexes. Carbohydrates that break down slowly, releasing glucose gradually into the bloodstream, have lower glycemic indexes.

The new term being used now to measure glycemic index in food is the glycemic load. The glycemic load provides a better indication of ideal food choice by measuring the total carbohydrate in a typical serving of the food and in a miniscule portion of 50 grams.

Proteins – The Building Blocks of Muscles

Since ancient times, protein was thought to be the nutrient responsible for strength and stamina. Writings about the first Olympic games in 776 BC tell of various animal meat, such as goat and deer, that the athletes ate before their competitions. In the report from the 1936 Olympics in Berlin, it was noted that the German athletes would eat over two pounds of meat per day. A pre-event meal often consisted of one or more steaks and several eggs. Slowly, research started to show the importance of carbohydrates and fat for energy production and total performance. Although carbohydrates are now known to be the muscle's primary fuel source, because fat provides the most concentrated storage form of energy for the body, protein is essential for anyone concerned about performance. How much of each you eat depends on how muscular you are and how much the measure of your body weight is derived from protein.

What is protein?

Protein is a macronutrient like carbohydrates and fat. All macronutrients contain carbon, oxygen and hydrogen molecules. Protein differs from carbohydrates and fats in that it also contains nitrogen, sulphur and some minerals. When 100 or more amino acids link together, a protein is formed. Proteins are made by following specific genetic code, so the amino acids are linked together in ways that turn on or off genes and codes for specific proteins.

Over 10,000 different proteins help make you who you are. The burning process of proteins involves 20 different amino acids. Of the 20 amino acids, none are considered essential because the body cannot produce them by themselves. Because the body needs a daily supply of these amino acids, protein is an essential nutrient that needs to be consumed daily. Everyone knows that protein is important for building muscles and for the repair of muscle fibers after exercise. That is why proteins in the body have passive, or essential, roles. including producing antibodies for the immune system; manufacturing hormones and enzymes that are involved in most reactions in your body; eating, digesting, and absorbing food; acting as a source of fuel when glycogen levels in the muscles are low; maximizing the transport of oxygen to tissue; and providing structure for muscles, tendons, ligaments, organs, bones, hair, skin and all other tissues.

You need to eat protein-containing foods daily to obtain your daily requirement for essential amino acids. About 90% of the protein you eat is broken down into amino acids and becomes part of the amino acids pool that our body draws upon when it needs to build or repair muscles and other tissues or to take care of any of the other roles that the amino acid plays. The body excretes the other 10%. Unlike carbohydrates and fats, which the body can store as glycogen or triglycerides specifically for use later, amino acids have no form of storage in the body, so it's important to have some protein every day. When you eat foods containing proteins, the protein molecule is broken down into the amino acids in your mouth and small intestines. Once the protein is broken into amino acids, three things can happen. The amino acids can convert into glucose, convert into triglycerides and be stored as body fat, or be released into the bloodstream as passive proteins or free amino acids to be used as energy.

When you eat enough proteins to cover your body's amino acids needs, your body is considered to be in protein equilibrium. However, if you don't eat enough protein, protein already inside your body, usually in the form of muscle, is broken down to fill the amino acids pool. If you consume more protein than your body needs, the excess protein acids are broken down further, with the nitrogen, ammonia, uric acid and cretin secreted in urine and the part of the amino acid remaining stored either as body fat or muscle. I recommend consuming one gram of protein per body weight each day for maximum muscle building and fat loss.

Protein Timing and Types

When to eat protein is also important for active individuals. There is some evidence that pre- and post-exercise meals containing some essential amino acids will result in increase muscle mass compared to the gains from training alone. For endurance athletes, a post-exercise meal containing essential amino acids is important for added strength gains. At this time, the best karma is to eat small amounts of proteins at each meal and consume proteins with carbohydrates immediately after a serious exercise session to help the muscles facilitate glycogen stores as quickly as possible.

Post-exercise protein recommendations suggest eating a ratio of proteins to carbohydrates of 1:3. What that means is that for every 3 grams of carbohydrates, you have one gram of protein. There are several sports bars and drinks designed to provide this combination of nutrients, or you can easily do it yourself with whole foods such as a turkey sandwich or a fruit smoothie with protein powder. Protein timing can also be important due to the speed of absorption and availability differences in the types of amino acids and hormonal responses that occur as a result of protein.

Fats

What is dietary fat? These fat inputs are referred to as lipids. Lipids come from the Greek word *lipose*, which means fat. Fat in food is an essential nutrient just like carbohydrates, protein, vitamin C, vitamin E, or any other essential nutrient. Fat is the most concentrated energy source of any macronutrients. It also necessitates the digestion and absorbs vitamins A, D, E, and K, along with hundreds of beneficial creatinols such as lycopin and lutin.

Fats also provide the body with essential fatty acids called linoleic and linolenic acids that help maintain the immune system and provide strong nails, shiny hair, and clear skin. Fatty acids produce hormones that affect everything from hunger and sex drive to your moods, but all fats are not created equal. There are good and bad fats that either help protect you from disease or increase your risk of chronic conditions. The so-called healthy fats are mono-unsaturated or poly-unsaturated fats. And the bad fats are the saturated fats and trans fats. When mono- or poly-unsaturated fats are substituted for saturated fats or trans fats in diets, they lower total blood cholesterol and triglycerides and raise healthy HDL cholesterol levels in the blood. They also improve insulin sensitivity and blood pressure. Saturated fats and trans fats, on the other hand, may promote heart disease, diabetes, certain cancers, and obesity because they raise LDL cholesterol levels. When trans fats get into the arteries, they elevate triglycerides and lower healthy HDL cholesterol levels.

The body can store unlimited amounts of fat. For most normal weight individuals, fat stores contain at least one hundred times more available energy as compared to stored carbohydrates. All of these stored triglycerides can be burned for fuel during exercise. However, the amount of fat versus carbohydrates burnt during exercise depends upon the duration and intensity of your workouts. A low-intensity fat oxidation provides a bulk of energy to the muscle, but as intensity increases, the percentage of carbohydrates oxidize for fuel increases. Once you reach 70% to 80% of your VO2 max, fat oxidation is limited and carbohydrates provide 70 to 80% of the energy. Compared to burning one glucose molecule for energy, fatty acids create nearly four times as much energy. However, fat oxidation requires more oxygen than carbohydrate oxidation, and when you start breathing hard, your ability to burn fat as fuel diminishes.

Aerobic training makes the body more efficient at burning fat as fuel by increasing the enzymes that are necessary to turn fatty acids into energy. This helps to spare carbohydrates, therefore enhancing endurance. An experienced marathon runner, for instance, will have the ability to burn more fat as fuel at the same percentage of VO2 max compared to an untrained individual.

Here are some examples of mono-unsaturated fats: olive oils, canola oils, peanut oils, nuts and avocados.

Here are some examples of poly-unsaturated fats, which include omega 3 and omega 6 fats. Omega 3 fats include: cold water fish, red herring, mackerel, salmon, sardines and tuna, flex seed, canola oil, and walnuts. Here are some examples of omega 6 fats: corn, safflower, sesame, soy and sunflower oils, nuts, and seeds.

Here are some examples of saturated fats: meats, poultry, butter, cheese, cream, whole milk, coconut, and processed foods such as cookies, crackers, chips, and other baked goods.

Here are some examples of trans fats: margarines, shortenings, packaged baked goods such as cookies, pastries, crackers, candies, snacks, French fries, and other fried foods.

Vitamins and Minerals Simplified

Vitamins and minerals are considered micronutrients because your body needs them in minute amounts. The foremost question on everyone's mind is probably whether you really need additional vitamins and minerals or if you are getting enough from eating food. Well, the basic answer is maybe. You see, there are many variables involved in meeting your daily vitamin and mineral requirements, and it's nearly impossible to give one answer that covers everyone's needs. What we will do is take a look at some of the variables so that you can decide if increasing your vitamin/mineral intake is warranted.

If any of these variables cause personal concern, there's a possibility that some additional vitamins and minerals may benefit you. So, let's look at these. There's a theory that faming soil is depleted of nutrients because of over-farming contributing to fruits and vegetables having less-than-optimum levels of nutrients. Extreme cooking of vegetables under a high temperature can significantly reduce the vitamin content. Cigarette smoking may contribute to a loss in calcium, along with vitamins B and C. Alcohol consumption may contribute towards losses in C and D vitamins. Coffee and caffeine may contribute towards losses in calcium and vitamins B and C.

Okay, let's recap a little bit. Vitamins and minerals are considered to be micronutrients. Minerals and non-organic vitamins are naturally grown on earth. Most vitamins are naturally-occurring organic compounds and can be found in plants. Some are derived from animal sources. Vitamin D is synthesized in the body when the skin is exposed to direct sunlight. Vitamin K is produced by macro-organisms in the digestive tract.

Vitamins can be classified as fat-soluble or water-soluble. Fat-soluble vitamins are vitamins A, D, E and K. Water-soluble vitamins are vitamins B and C. Fat-soluble vitamins are stored in the body for an extended period of time, therefore giving them a higher chance of over dosage. Water-soluble vitamins are flushed out of the body throughout the day; therefore, there's less chance of toxicity.

Vitamins themselves do not provide energy; rather, they assist the body with optimizing counter functions. Synthesized soluble vitamins such as vitamins A and D may have the most risk for toxicity. In most cases, you would have to work hard to reach the safe upper limit of vitamin and mineral consumption. Sensible use of vitamin- and mineral-fortified foods won't put people at risk. The importance of vitamins and minerals for your overall health and fitness performance should be glaringly apparent. Macronutrients assist in processes throughout the body and directly impact your ability to exercise, recover, and form new muscle tissues and a strong skeletal system. Does this necessarily mean that you need to run out and start hyper-dosing on vitamins and minerals? No, this just means that you need to pay close attention to what you are eating. A deficiency in any one vitamin or mineral may mean that some biological process somewhere in the body may not be working at its optimal level. This could ultimately hinder your performance.

Dieticians and nutritionists are to some degree opposed to vitamin and mineral supplementation. On the other hand, fitness enthusiasts believe that more is better. This information isn't meant to sway your thinking in either direction, only to give you a reasonable perspective on the subject matter so you will come to your own conclusion. Since there are so many variables involved with consuming and maintaining adequate levels of micronutrients, it makes sense for some people to use additional vitamins and minerals as an insurance policy against deficiencies. Considering that those concerned with their fitness want to ensure that their bodies are functioning at optimal levels at all times, any simple biological process that is not working in its full potential may ultimately lead to hindered performance.

This prospect is unacceptable for those wanting to better their athletic performance under certain conditions. Even those looking for average results may need a little help consuming the RDA (recommended daily allowance) of vitamins and minerals, especially if they experience or are exposed to poor dietary habits, excessive stress, smoking, drinking, and living in areas with elevated levels of pollution. Always remember that there is no cure, capsule, or supplement that can take the place of a sensible nutrition plan and hard training. Nutritional products should only be used to enhance an already sound regimen and, in this manner, they might help to optimize your nutritional plan and performance by guarding against nutrition deficiency.

Individualize Your Diet

Making dietary changes doesn't mean giving up your favorite foods or completely changing your lifes Simply moderate how much of your favorite foods you eat by having them less often and then learn how to make healthier substitutions.

Advanced Weight-Loss Technique

As a doctor concerned about the lack of awareness and confusion people have over the best way to lose weight, I want to help clear up some common weight-loss myths. In the 1990s, we were told that all fat was bad for us. Now carbs are being blamed for America's increasing waistline. Even some athletes have fallen into the low carb trap. I urge you not to make this same mistake. If you want to lose weight, build muscle, have tons of energy, and improve your skin and sex drive, you need to eat carbs. It's true, carbs are good for you. You just need to know when and how to eat them.

First, let's dispel some myths about low-carb diets such as the Atkins diet. It is estimated that nearly 60 million Americans have tried to avoid carbohydrate-rich foods like bread, pasta, and cereal. Even Burger King is cashing in on this trend by selling their bunless burger. Still, the average person's weight in this country continues to increase.

What is going wrong? For starters, low-carb diets do not work long-term because they contain too many calories. They also require you to avoid carbohydrates for the rest of your life, which quickly leaves most people feeling deprived and unsatisfied. Eating should be pleasurable, not stressful. Even worse, low-carbohydrate diets can wreck your metabolism and damage your health. Traditionally, a low-carb diet can ban fruits and certain vegetables. It just doesn't make sense to deny your body these foods. Fruits protect against cancer, hypertension, and heart disease. Getting healthy is not just about losing weight, it's about gaining health. For years, I helped members of Fitness Concepts lose fat, build muscle, and improve their performance by altering between days of eating normal amounts of carbohydrates and days of limited carbohydrate consumption.

This method produced amazing results because it was based on real science, not marketing hype by the diet industry. Not to mention that I also used it to win a first-place title in every different weight class in body building. When I started my business, Fitness Concepts, in 1999, I started seeing clients who dieted and exercised regularly but could not lose weight. They didn't realize that a slow metabolism was derailing their efforts. That's when I decided to create a plan that could be as effective as a program I developed for them. So I developed a program that was called the Carb Cycling Diet. The key to carb cycling is learning how to exploit the two important bodily processes that determine how you look and feel, anabolism and catabolism.

Anabolism is a process through which your body builds muscle. Catabolism is a process through which your body burns fat. Low-carb diets focus only on changing your metabolism. They do not help you build muscle by alternating between low-carb and high-carb days, by using a program like the Carb Cycling Diet that has helped my clients to get the lean, strong bodies they have always wanted. They also enjoy the luxury of eating the foods they love as long as they eat them at the right time. It takes a little discipline at first, but it is ultimately far easier and healthier than restricting diets like Atkins.

During normal carb days, I recommend eating between 350 to 400 grams of carbohydrates. That's about what you probably are already eating. Keep in mind that you should focus on eating every kind of carbs from whole grains, fruits and vegetables. The only refined carbs are sugar and processed white flour. On limited carb days, do not eat any foods containing sugar or white flour. Try to keep your carbs under 100 grams per day. You should never starve yourself or feel hungry. Even on loaded carb days, this may sound tricky; it's not. Counting carbs is pretty easy once you get the hang of it, plus the small extra effort will bring you a huge payoff.

If you combine carb cycling with exercise, you will protect yourself from age-related illnesses such as osteoarthritis, cardiovascular disease, and even cancer. You'll also look and feel great.

How To Manipulate Your Nutrient Intake To Maximize Fat Loss

I like the concept called carbohydrate cycling. This is a secret that bodybuilders have been using for years to drop every bit of fat from their bodies and to get a hard, ripped physique. You don't need to be a bodybuilder, though. This secret will work just as well for the average person. This is a short-term diet strategy that consists of three principles; cutting way back on fat intake, limiting carbohydrate consumption, and increasing protein consumption.

Cutting back on fats is obvious. Get rid of butter or fatty foods from your diet. Remove any skin or visible fat from the meats. Pretty simple stuff. In addition to dropping fats from your diet, you will want to limit carbohydrates, which will suppress the release of insulin. One of the effects of insulin is to increase the uptake and storage of dietary fats. By limiting carbohydrates, you choke off the body's supply of insulin, thus increasing fat loss.

The additional extra protein in your diet is to help spare your existing muscle. One of the downsides to limiting carbohydrate intake is that after about 3 to 5 days, your body will enter a state of ketosis. This happens when the muscles no longer have a source of glycogen, or stored carbohydrates, to burn as fuel. The body will then look at alternate sources of energy, and because there's not sufficient protein available, your body will start using muscle tissue for fuel. Following is my seven-step guide to manipulating carbohydrates to promote maximum fat loss while maintaining your existing muscle mass. This guide assumes you are eating six meals a day already and drinking lots of water. It also assumes you are exercising daily.

Step number one – Think low carbs, not high fat. Forget about diets that have you striving for zero carbohydrates while still eating plenty of high-fat foods like whole eggs, fatty beef, and cheese. The winning strategy is to limit carbohydrates and fat or make lean proteins your key ingredients to stave off muscle loss.

Step number two – Take the number of carbohydrates you would normally eat and divide it by two. A normal, 200-pound male will usually eat about 500 grams of carbohydrates daily. Follow this plan by eating one-half of the usual carbohydrates per day, or 250 grams for one day. Next, slash that reduced total in half once more, or 125 grams, and stick with that lowered carbohydrate intake for two more days, spreading carbohydrate consumption evenly over the day.

Step number three – Eat your carbohydrates before and after exercise. During days four and five, you will keep your carbohydrate intake at reduced levels. Eat carbohydrates only before and after you exercise, keeping your carbohydrates intake even throughout the day. This will help to spare your muscles while depleting carbohydrates in the body and kicking your insulin mechanism into high gear.

Step number four – Slice carbs to the bone. Now that you have depleted your muscles of glycogen, you can really push the envelope for two days. This is the hardest part of the seven-step plan as your glycogen levels will be so low that you will have very low energy. Cut your carbohydrate intake back to 75 grams for the next two days. Try to eat the majority of the carbohydrates before exercise to give you the energy you need. For the rest of the day, the only carbohydrates you get should come from veggies.

Step number five – Switch it up for one glorious day. When you are on a low-carbohydrate diet, your body will adapt, which will slow down your metabolism and your rate of calories being burned. You can treat your body by switching things up for one day and keeping metabolism and fat burning in high gear. Increase your carbohydrate intake by 80% of what's normal for you. This is 400 grams for the above-referenced 200-pound man. This increase will fuel your body and keep your metabolism high while providing you with much-needed energy at this point. Don't forget to increase your protein. During your reduced carbohydrates, you will need additional protein to keep your body from using your muscles as fuel. Follow the schedule below for protein intake and avoid this problem.

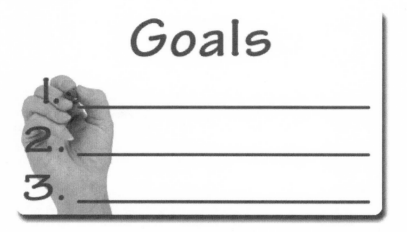

Day one – 1 gram of protein per pound of body weight

Days two and day three – 1.2 grams of protein per pound of body weight

Days four and day five – 1.6 grams of protein per pound of body weight

Days six and day seven – 1.8 grams of protein per pound of body weight

Day eight – 1 gram of protein per pound of body weight

Step number seven – Rest and repeat. Repeat the previous six steps up to three times, and then take a one-week break. After seven days of this plan, there's no doubt that you will reach your weight loss goals. To recap, here's the total plan.

Day one – 250 grams of carbohydrates and 1 gram of protein per pound of body weight

Days two and three – 125 grams of carbohydrates and 1.2 grams of protein per pound of body weight

Days four and five – 125 grams of carbohydrates, one-half before and one-half after your workout, and 1.6 grams of protein per pound of body weight

Days six and seven – 75 grams of carbohydrates and 1.8 grams of protein per pound of body weight

Day eight – 400 grams of carbohydrates and 1 gram of protein per pound of body weight

You also want to make sure you eat 6 meals per day, drink at least 64 ounces of water per day, and exercise daily.

More Advanced Weight Loss Tips and Tricks.

Here I will list 10 more of the most hyper-effective fat-burning tactics that I've discovered from nearly 20 years in the bodybuilding and personal training and coaching industries. These are some of the same techniques I've used to hit 3 to 4% of body fat for competition and see a regular 9% body fat composition all year round, year after year, without difficultly. If you already have all of the basics covered and you want to incinerate every last bit of fat, then this is good information for you.

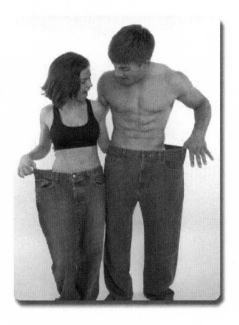

Strategy number one – Do cardio daily. If you progress and increase your cardio as needed up to as much as 30 to 45 minutes per day, 6 to 7 days per week for 8 to 12 weeks, you will get so lean, you'll kick yourself for not realizing it was that simple. Now, I would not necessarily recommend starting with this amount of exercise, particularly if you are a beginner. However, if you already exercise but are not really satisfied with your fat loss, I highly recommend that you slowly and progressively increase your cardio to a point where you are doing it daily. Every time I give this advice, I always hear lots of whining and complaining. Why is everybody so cardio-phobic? Why do people keep fighting the daily exercise concept when they've tried everything else and they still can't get as lean as they want to be?

Now, here's what I hear, "But Sam, isn't 20 minutes, 3 days a week the solution? But Sam, doesn't too much cardio burn up muscle? But Sam, doesn't weight training boost the metabolism more than cardio? But Sam, isn't long aerobic cardio out and anaerobic and HRT cardio in?" People have plenty of thoughts. The irony is that they start out with all of these buts and at the same time they're stuck and they can't figure out why they are not losing those last few pockets of seriously annoying body fat.

If you want to get really lean, get off your butt and do what it takes to get the job done, not what the trend of the month says. Let me ask you a question. When you read books and articles or courses about the world's best bodybuilding and fitness model, what is the common denominator you see in nearly 100% of the pre-contest preparation programs? You have cardio daily in the 30- to 45-minutes range, and some even do cardio up to an hour a day or more during the pre-contest period. If you want to know why frequent cardio burns more fat, go back and re-read the previous sections.

By the way, daily cardio is not something you do all the time. This is a strategy that you progressively build up to and use for short periods in order to hit a peak, break plateaus, and shed the last couple pounds of fat. Doing daily cardio year around leads to aerobic adaptation. Cardio must be cycled just like all other factors related to fat loss.

You increase cardio during periods when fat loss is desired and reduce cardio during periods when maintenance is desired. By the way, not having enough time is not a valid excuse. I know many people who get up at 5:00 in the morning to workout because it's the only way they can fit it into their schedule. It's never an issue of time; it's always an issue of willingness and priorities. Are you willing to do what it takes to get the results you want? Are you willing to make weight loss a priority in your life? That's the only real question you have to answer.

Strategy number two – Do your cardio first thing in the morning on an empty stomach. Fast, early morning cardio is still controversial in academic circles, and some people are concerned that it might be too catabolic and you may break down muscle along with the fat. However, my experience and some research has shown that while there are risks, fast and early morning cardio does work, and the potential benefits outweigh those risks. But don't take my word for it. Examine the facts. Test yourself carefully, monitoring your body composition and lean mass, and decide for yourself if early morning cardio will work for you. The argument in favor of fast, early morning cardio goes something like this:

After getting eight to twelve hours of sleep overnight, your body stores of glycogen are depleted, and you burn more fat when glycogen is low. Secondly, eating causes a release of insulin, which interferes with the metabolism of body fat. Less insulin is present in the morning; therefore, more fat is burned when cardio is done in the morning. Third, there are less carbohydrates in the bloodstream when you wake up after an overnight fast. With less glucose available, you burn more fat. Fourth, if you eat immediately before a workout, you have to burn off what you just ate first before tapping into the stored body fat. Fifth, when you do cardio in the morning, your metabolism stays elevated for a period of time after the workout is over. If you do cardio in the evening, you burn calories during the session, but you fail to take advantage of the after-burn effect because your metabolism break drops automatically as soon as you fall asleep.

Strategy number three – Reduce your carbs, but don't cut them all out and don't stay on low carbs too long. As you know, I'm not a big fan of very low-carbohydrates diets or ketotanic diets. Although they have worked for many people, most people report that they make you feel like crap. You get brain fog, you lose muscle along with the fat, and your training intensity suffers from lack of muscle glycogen. You are on a cyclic glycogenic diet. Low carbs and high activity don't go well together. There are real side effects of very low carbohydrate–diet, or VLCD, that few people think of because it requires a long-term perspective and most people are caught up in a short-term solution. For the average non–bodybuilder, it is very difficult to permanently keep weight off if it's lost through VLCD. VLCD will set you up for a big rebound. Bodybuilders often use VLCDs successfully before a contest, but bodybuilders are extreme athletes with incredible discipline and willpower. I know bodybuilders who are so hard core that they can eat nothing but tuna fish out of the can for twelve weeks, then go back to a normal balanced diet like it's no problem, no big thing. That's a rare feat. Lots of people lose weight on very low-carbohydrates diets, but few keep it off. I've seen people go on massive uncontrollable binges of donuts, pizza and then end up gaining 30 pounds in less than seven days after coming off a low-carbohydrate diet.

Low-carbohydrate diets are not the long-term solution for fat loss. To use one successfully without gaining everything back, you have to know what you are doing, and you must be extremely disciplined. Even then, you should consider low-carbohydrate diets as a last-chance diet or short-term peak diet that is fraught with side effects and disadvantages.

A balanced diet containing a wide variety of foods, including about 40% to 50% of calories from vegetables, fruits, natural starches, and 100% whole grains is almost always the best way to permanently lose fat and is the way almost everyone should start. This is sometimes referred to as a base line diet. All you have to do is exercise, eat the right types of foods and eat less than you burn each day, and you will lose fat. Also, if you master the basics, you'll reach the advanced stage. I have to admit that despite the potential pitfalls, low-carb, high-protein diets can help accelerate fat loss even more at the advanced stage.

Almost every competitive bodybuilder I've ever met uses some variation of the reduced-carb diet. A low carb diet also alleviates water retention and gives us a hard, dry look. However, there's a right and wrong way to do a low-carb diet. Here are the seven advanced bodybuilding secrets to using a low-carb diet successfully.

Number one – Don't cut out all carbs, just reduce them to a moderate level so carbs and proteins are balanced and carbs are not the predominant macronutrients. You don't have to cut down to next to nothing to get low-carb diet benefits. Don't eat a lot of carbs at night, but do eat natural starches and grains early in the day after your workouts.

Number two – Don't stay on a reduced-carb diet for more than 12 to 16 weeks. Always go back to a more balanced diet, which is healthier and more maintainable over long periods of time.

Number three – Take a periodic carb-up day or re-feed day. This will help you to stop your metabolism from slowing down, keep your thyroid functioning optimally, and maintain your energy levels.

Number four – Raise your lean protein and healthy fats. Traditional bodybuilding and fat-reducing wisdom that says you should eat 1 gram of protein per pound of body weight. This is good advice for someone just starting to establish good habits and a baseline nutrition plan. For example, a 172-pound man would consume 172 grams of protein, which equals approximately 30 grams per meal spread over 5 to 6 meals.

However, reducing your carbohydrates can give some metabolic and hormonal advantage for fat loss when it is done properly and not taken on an extreme. When you start bringing your carbs down, something has to go, which often means that your calories will drop too low and you will lose your primary energy source. As a result, the something that "goes" will likely be lean protein and healthy fats, even though many mainstream low-carb diets like Atkins are actually high-fat, very low-carb diets. Competitive bodybuilders usually keep the fats at a moderate 20% to 30% of total calories while eating extremely large amounts of proteins, sometimes as much as 40% or even 50% of their total calories. This appears to be an obscene amount of protein. However, high-protein diets are one of the secrets that bodybuilders use to get ripped and speed up their metabolism.

Number five – Get total clarity or purpose. To get super lean, you have to decide exactly what you want so you can lock in on your goal the way a guided missile locks onto his target. The great Napoleon Hill called it definiteness of purpose. Most of us simply know it as having goals. Let's say you want to gain muscle and lose fat. That's a goal, but it's a poor goal because it lacks clarity. One of the biggest reasons people fail to move up to their mass levels is because they can't decide what they want, so they become victims of flip flop syndrome. Imagine a captain gives no commands and just allows his ship to float around careless, drifting wherever the current takes it, or that he gives instructions to his crew that sound like this: "Go east! No, go west. No, go east! No, go west again." Ridiculous, right? But this is exactly what you are doing when you have no specific goals at all or when you want to gain muscle one day and lose fat the next.

You have to make up your mind. I made up my mind with tremendous extra power. You must choose a definite course, make a clear-cut definite decision, and follow through with action in one specific direction. There must be no doubt. If on one hand, you want to get ripped, but on the other you are worried about losing all of your muscle, you are subconsciously sabotaging yourself every time you workout.

Number six – Eat five meals a day for women or six meals a day for men, or just forget about it. Most fitness-conscious people already understand the importance of meal frequency but figure they can get by with three square meals. Comparing three square meals to six meals a day is like comparing a porcelain tow boat to a u-boat. Yes, you can get some results with three square meals, but you'll never get anywhere near your maximum potential, and the results you do get will take a lot longer.

The benefits of frequent eating include a faster metabolism, higher energy levels, less storage of body fat, reduced hunger and cravings, steadier blood sugar and insulin levels, more calories that can be used for muscle growth, and better absorption and utilization of nutrients. If you want to move to the advanced level and get super lean, you have to take advantage of every weapon in your fat-burning arsenal, which includes five or six meals a day or, as Al Pacino would say, just forget about it.

Number seven – Go easy on those protein bars and meal replacement shakes; focus on real food instead. My clients just hate me when I take away their cookies-and-cream protein bars and chocolate shakes, but when they are eating only one or two full meals per day and using four or five meal replacements and wondering why they are not getting leaner, I have to give them a lecture on thermogenic effects of whole foods versus liquid calories and protein bars. If you want to get lean, don't drink too many of your calories, and lay off those bars to determine the effect of whole food to help you get leaner. Use supplements for convenience once in a while, not as a primary source of your calories.

HIIT The Fat

HIIT, which stands for High-Intensity Interval Training, is a technique of alternating short periods, usually 30 or 60 seconds, of very high-intensity cardio with short periods of low intensity cardio High-intensity interval training workouts should last only 15 to 25 minutes total. HIIT has received a lot of press lately as being superior to steady exercise. In some ways, it is superior. HIIT burns a lot of calories during the workout but where it really shines is after a workoutHere's an example of 21 minutes of HIIT workouts on the lifecycle bike.

Level three – 5 minutes

Level five – 1 minute

Level four – 1 minute

Level six – 1 minute

Level four – 1 minute

Level seven – 1 minute

Level four – 1 minute

Level eight – 1 minute

Level four – 1 minute

Level nine – 1 minute

Level four – 1 minute

Level 10 – 1 minute

Level three – 5 minute

This is just an example of a course you might take. You need to adjust the workout based on your fitness level, so you can adjust the duration of each interval, the number of levels (or duration of the workout) and the difficulty levels. You can perform similar workouts on almost any piece of cardio equipment. HIIT is often thought of as a superior fat-burning method, but it really depends what you are comparing it to. When compared to low-intensity, long-duration cardio as it frequently is, HIIT wins hands down. Low-intensity cardio, like casual walking, is never the best way to lose fat, except for beginners who are not physically prepared for high intensity yet. If your intensity is moderate to moderate/high and your health level is ready for long duration workouts, you are likely to burn more fat with this approach than you would in a 15- to 20-minute non-HIIT workout. Of course this is relative   to exercise, intensity and duration. However, if the intensity is high enough, you can get a very efficient workout in a relatively short period of time using HIIT.

HIIT works, but I should warn you: it is not stable. What is most important for fat loss is that you burn a lot of calories with moderate- to high-intensity cardio. My best advice is to use both forms of cardio training, relying on HIIT when you are short on time or when you have hit a plateau on moderate, long-duration cardio for an extended period of time. Remember that eventually, your body adapts to everything.

Strategy Number Nine – Do all of your cardio harder. Here is an idea that might shatter every paradigm you ever heard about cardio training. As we just talked about, HIIT is very trendy these days. So, if you are trying to lose fat and you are wondering whether you should do short-duration, high-intensity or long-duration, low–intensity cardio, the answer might be neither. The most effective workout is long–duration, high–intensity cardio, provided that you are healthy, you have received your doctor's approval to perform high-intensity exercise, and you have already built a substantial base level of aerobic fitness. You can gradually push up your intensity to the highest level that you can hold steady for the entire duration of your cardio workout, whether that is 20 minutes, 30 minutes, or even 45 minutes. In other words, no coasting. Put the cell phones and the magazines away and do a real, killer cardio workout. Your body will get leaner by the day. Of course, intensity and duration are inversely related. So, technically, you can't do long durations of high intensity, but what we are talking about is to do as high intensity as you can for as long as you can. The proper name for this type of cardio workout is moderately high-intensity cardio.

Strategy number ten – Split your daily routine. We all know that exercise increases your metabolic rate way after exercise is performed, especially if you're using HIIT training and anaerobic training. Well, if you are going to try to lose the maximum amount of fat possible, and if you had the time to do it right, I would definitely either do HIIT training in the morning and anaerobic or weight training exercise in the evening or vice versa. This way, you have elevated your metabolism pretty much all day and all night long.

Weight-Loss Diets

Losing weight means losing body fat. And you can lose body fat 2 ways: by limiting the intake of high-fat foods or by consuming fat-burning foods. Either of these will not only improve one's metabolism, but it will also allow him to eat more food for his calorie expenditure because fats have more than twice the calories per gram as proteins (which contain 4 calories per gram) and carbohydrates.

Low-Fat Diet

A low-fat diet involves intake of food that has few fat calories instead of those with high fat calories. This type of diet is ideal to prevent someone from being obese. Thus, this is advisable for those who do not yet suffer from obesity and want to avoid experiencing it. Most parents prefer this type of diet for their children due to the fear that they might grow obese. Below is a diet suggestion for general good health or for dietary treatment. Foods are categorized according to low-fat foods (allowed to consume) and high-fat foods (prohibited from consuming):

Fat-Burning Diet

A fat-burning diet is about burning unwanted fat calories that are stored in the body. Certain foods and eating habits can be used to accelerate fat-burning, either directly by promoting the meltdown of the body's stored fats or indirectly by modifying our energy use. These foods include:

Protein-Rich Foods – These foods below significantly increase the metabolic rate (the pace at which we use food as fuel), creating heat and burning many more calories than carbohydrates or fat.

- **Fat-Burning Protein Foods**
  - **Lean Meat:** Beef, lamb, veal, venison, rabbit, hare, offal

  - **Poultry:** Chicken, turkey, pheasant, grouse, guinea fowl

  - **Fish:** Cod, haddock, plaice, sole, coley, whiting, mackerel, trout, salmon

  - **Shellfish:** Scallops, shrimp, prawns, lobster, crab, scampi, cockles, mussels, winkles, whelks, abalone

  - **Cheese:** Mainly low-fat cottage cheese, use reduced-fat versions of hard cheeses, such as Cheddar, in moderation

- **Eggs**
- **Soya products**
- **Negative-Calorie Foods –** More calories are needed to break down, digest, and assimilate these foods than they supply. Eating mainly negative-calorie foods is said to reduce weight three times faster than fasting and to reduce body weight by an average of 0.5 kg (1 lb) per day.

- o Negative Calorie Foods include:**Vegetables:** Asparagus, aubergine (eggplant), beetroot, broccoli, Brussels sprouts, cabbage, carrots, cauliflower, celeriac, celery, chicory, Chinese cabbage (pak choi, bok choi), cress, dandelion leaves, endive, fennel, globe artichokes, green beans, leeks, lettuce, mangetouts (snow peas), mooli (daikon or Japanese radish), mushrooms, okra (ladies' fingers), onions, radishes, seaweed, spinach, squash, swede, tomatoes, turnips

- o **Fruits:** Apples, apricots, bananas, blackberries, blackcurrants, blueberries, boysenberries, cherries, clementines, cranberries, damsons, figs, gooseberries, grapefruit, grapes, greengages, guavas, kiwi fruit, kumquat, loquat, lychees, mandarins, mangos, medlars, melons, mulberries, nectarines, oranges, papaya, peaches, pears, persimmons, pineaaple, plums, pomegranate, prickly pear, raspberries, redcurrants, satmusas, star fruit, strawberries, whitecurrants

- **Nuts:** Almonds, barcelona nuts, Brazil nuts, chestnuts, coconuts, filberts, hazelnuts, macademias, peanuts, pine nuts, pistachios, walnuts

Low-GI (Glycaemic Index) Carbohydrate Foods – These foods help us to burn the food at our disposal rather than storing it as fat. Examples include:

- **Breads:** Multigrain breads (white and brown), heavy fruit breads

- **Grains and Breakfast Cereals:** Brown rice, wild rice, other whole grains,   tabbouleh,   pearl   barley,   whole wheat pasta, oats, porridge,   unsweetened muesli, high-fiber wheat bran cereal

- **Vegetables:** Sweet potato, okra mushrooms, legumes (peas, beans), broccoli, artichokes, aubergines

- **Fruits:** Apples, pears, oranges, mandarins, grapefruit, bananas

- **Other:** Honey, jam, Soya milk and its products

CHAPTER 4
The Proper Exercises

It is an accepted fact that exercise is an important part of any successful weight-loss plan. Every muscle in your body can burn calories, so the more you work them, the more calories they can burn. So, don't just depend on dieting to lose weight. Move that body by doing some exercises to achieve that trim body you have always dreamed about.

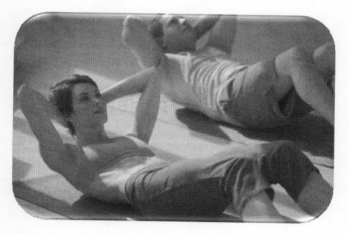

Deep Breathing

Although deep breathing alone can not eradicate the excess fat hanging by your belly or legs, it will make you calmer, reduce your stress, and give you increased energy to use throughout the day.

- **When to do it:** Practice deep breathing exercises upon waking in the morning, before going to sleep at night, and at least once during the day.

- **How to do it:** Stand comfortably, or lie down if you happen to be on a bed – whatever's more comfortable and convenient for you. Take a deep breath, drawing your breath in slowly over a count of 5 seconds. Fill your lungs with fresh air as full as possible. Hold your breath for 20 seconds or for as long as you can without straining yourself, and then breathe out again very slowly to a count of 10. Repeat a total of 15 times.

Walking

Walking is great exercise to lose weight. Moreover, it does not require any expertise or equipment, and you can do it free of charge anytime you feel like it. However, to be beneficial, you should do it regularly.

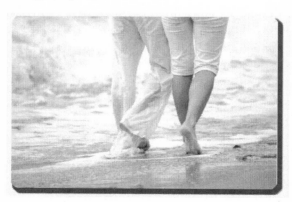

- **When to do it:** Make walking a daily habit or at least 3-5 times a week depending on your schedule.

- **How to do it:** Before you start walking, do some warm-up stretching exercises. Stretch only as far as you feel comfortable so as not to injure yourself. Start with a modest goal, like 15 to 20 minutes at a leisurely pace. Gradually extend the duration and the speed. Walk up one or two gentle slopes. Your walk should be comprised of three segments: warm-up, exercise pace and cool-down.

Doing it Right

- Walk with your chin up and your shoulders held slightly back.

- The heel of your foot should touch the ground first. Roll your weight forward.

- Swing your arms as you walk.

- To avoid stiff or sore muscles or joints, start gradually. Over several weeks, begin walking faster, going further, and walking for longer periods of time.

- Walk on soft ground.

- Quench yourself – drink 8-10 ounces of water for every 20 minutes of the activity.

Significance

The more you walk, the better you will feel. Plus, walking also uses calories; thus, burning fat. Its benefits include giving you more energy, making you feel good, helping you relax, reducing stress, helping you sleep better, toning your muscles, helping you control your appetite, and increasing the number of calories your body uses.

To lose weight, it's more important to walk for longer periods of time than at quicker speeds. Walking at a moderate pace yields longer workouts with less soreness – leading to more miles crossed and more calories spent on a regular basis.

Aerobics Training

Cardio exercise can be loosely defined as an existing activity of sufficient intensity to strengthen the cardio respiratory system when repeated consistently. One of the virtues of cardio exercise is that a wide range of activities meet these criteria, from walking to bicycling to work; just about anyone can find at least one form of cardio exercise he or she enjoys.

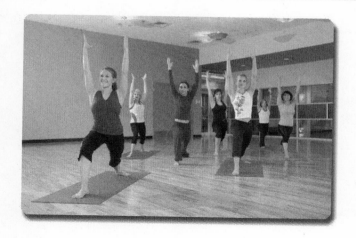

You can also make cardio training fun by purposely taking advantage of a variety of offers through cross training, that is, by routinely practicing two or more cardio activities. The benefits of cardio exercise are wide-ranging. Perhaps its most important benefit is that it burns a large amount of calories. Cardio exercise causes the body to shed excess fat and to keep it off.

Cardio exercise not only makes us look better and feel better about ourselves, but it also greatly reduces our risk of various health problems that are related to being overweight, such as diabetes, high blood pressure, certain cancers, and stroke. Regular cardio exercise has also been known to reduce stress, increase performance in everyday activities, improve sleep and even improve memory and cognitive functions. In short, if you are not getting cardio exercise, you are not really living.

Guidelines for Cardio Exercises

Before beginning any kind of cardio exercise regimen, you should consult with your physician and have a physical examination to clear you of any healthy risks.

The three large, fundamental variables of cardio exercise are frequency, duration, and intensity. Together, the frequency and duration of a workout determine your time commitment to your cardio exercise. For the average person, the course to achieve optimum body composition and basic cardio respiratory fitness with a minimum amount of cardio exercise is to manipulate the intensity of your cardio workouts in the most effective way possible.

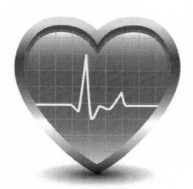

Exercise intensity refers to the rate at which your body is currently producing energy in relation to the maximum rate your body is able to produce energy for a specific activity. For example, suppose you were running five miles an hour. If you increase your pace just slightly to 5.1 miles an hour, your body is producing a little more energy and is therefore working at a higher intensity. Intensity is important because it is the primary determination of how your body adapts to exercise. At a certain intensity level, your body responds over time in such a way as to be found better able to train at the same intensity level. The more time you spend at that level, the more pronounced these adaptations become up to a limit. So it is important to know which training intensities are connected to which result. Once you have this knowledge, you can exercise at different intensities to get the results you seek.

The most practical way to measure and control intensity during a cardio workout is by body awareness. There are specific sensory tubes or body signals associated with each level of exercise intensity. You can use these to perform each type of cardio workout at the appropriate intensity and get the best results from your efforts. Use the following information for guidance:

Aerobic Intensity: In aerobic intensity, your breathing is elevated but controlled. You could speak one full sentence without gasping.

Threshold intensity: In threshold intensity, the effort feels comfortably hard. If you pick up the pace even a little bit, you will start to suffer.

Spent intensity: In spent intensity, you feel you are moving at the fastest pace you can maintain for a designated interval, usually 10 to 60 seconds.

There are many degrees of intensity; the above are just three general intensity ranges that you want to target in your workouts. In the aerobic intensity range, the aerobic energy system is trained. At threshold intensity, the first anaerobic system, primarily called anaerobic, causes restraint. At spent intensity, the second anaerobic system that creates the prospect system is trained. Each leads to its own set of beneficial adaptations, so your program should include all of them. Let's look at them one by one.

Aerobic Intensity

In aerobic metabolism, oxygen is used to break down primarily fatty acids and carbohydrates to release energy. An aerobic system produces harmless byproducts of carbon dioxide, water, and heat. For this reason, and because it is a supplier of its own energy, aerobic intensity is a great option. Aerobic intensity exercise can continue for long periods of time, especially in a well-conditioned individual. But because aerobic metabolism is relatively slow, this energy system is inadequate to support extremely high-intensity efforts. An intensive aerobic exercise results in many positive adaptations. It strengthens the heart and entire cardio respiratory system, not only benefiting your overall health but also enhancing performance in every form of exercise and any life activity you can name. Aerobic conditioning is truly the foundation of fitness.

Aerobic intensity exercise also increases your endurance so you can sustain activity for longer periods of time. It does this by increasing your body's fat-burning efficiency and glucose-storage capacity. Aerobic intensity exercises are also an excellent means of improving body composition because of the rate of fat-burning pieces in the middle of its intensity range and also because aerobic intensity exercise can be maintained much longer than exercise of higher intensity. The overall calorie-burning potential is greater with aerobic intensity exercise.

Threshold intensity

In threshold intensity anaerobic glycol sis exercises, glucose is broken down for energy without the use of oxygen.

This process is faster than aerobic metabolism, so it can support high-intensity efforts. However, anaerobic glycol sis produces metabolic waste products that can inhibit muscle contraction, resulting in exhaustion. The aerobics system can use these waste products as fuels for one exercise intensity process. Certain threshold wastes are produced faster than they are used. These wastes can accumulate in the muscles, which begin to burn and feel heat, and pretty soon you'll be working out at a near threshold.

Threshold intensity also carries significant benefits to begin with. It simply enhances the cardiovascular benefits that come from aerobic training and also enhances positive changes in your body composition, which results in being even more efficient than aerobics training because calories are burned faster at threshold intensity than aerobic intensity. For most serious exercisers and athletes, threshold intensity training greatly enhances the body's ability to recover between hard efforts in a workout or competition. This allows you to do a more advanced workout and get a more pronounced effect from it.

Spent intensity

Spent intensity is the second anaerobic energy system that creates a fast system to fuel maximum and near-maximum efforts such as heavy lifting. Spent intensity relies on cretin phosphate, of which only tiny amounts are stored in the muscle, so this energy system cannot support efforts lasting longer than 15 seconds. Spent intensity workouts burn more calories per minute than all workouts of lesser intensity. They are also an excellent supplement to strength training because they condition the same energy system and develop the same muscle fibers.

Aerobic Exercises

The word *aerobic* literally means "with oxygen" or "in the presence of oxygen." Aerobic exercise is any activity that uses large muscle groups, can be maintained continuously for a long period of time and is rhythmic in nature.

Aerobic exercises utilize oxygen as the major fuel for sustaining activity for relatively long periods. In general, aerobic exercises are those activities that require large muscle work, elevate the heart rate to between 60 percent and 80 percent of maximal heart rate, are continuous in nature, and are of 15 to 60 minutes in duration. An aerobically-fit individual can work longer and more vigorously, while also achieving a quicker recovery at the end of the aerobic session.

Types of Aerobic Exercises

Aerobic exercises fall into two categories:

- **Low- to Moderate-Impact Exercises** – These include walking, swimming, stair climbing, step classes, rowing, and cross-country skiing. Nearly anyone in reasonable health can engage in some low- to moderate-impact exercise. Brisk walking burns as many calories as jogging for the same distance and poses less risk for injury to muscle and bone.

- **High-Impact Exercises** – Activities that belong to this group include running, dance exercise, tennis, racquetball, and squash. High-impact exercises should be performed only every alternate day. People who are overweight, elderly, out of condition, or have an injury or other medical problem should do them even less frequently.

Some Aerobic Exercises

1. Walking

Walking is a popular form of exercise because it requires little in terms of equipment or facilities. Walking an extra 20 minutes each day will burn off 7 pounds of body fat per year. Longer, moderately-paced daily walks are best for losing weight.

2. Jogging/Running

With jogging or running, an individual is able to cover greater distances in a shorter period of time. Therefore, greater numbers of calories can be burned.

3. Choreographed Aerobic Exercise

Choreographed aerobic dance is a very popular form of exercise throughout the world. Aerobic dance helps in toning up the muscles of the body.

4. Step Aerobics

Step aerobics incorporates the use of a step or bench that is typically about one foot wide, three feet long, and about six inches high. Instructors use many moves that require participants to step up and down from the platform. This way, the activity will not be boring or tiring, but will be lively and motivating.

5. Water Aerobics

Water aerobics incorporates a variety of movements from both swimming and land aerobics to develop vigorous routines that are aerobic in nature. It utilizes the resistance to movement that water creates to elevate heart rates and helps in losing weight.

6. Swimming

Swimming is a very popular form of regular exercise. Due to the resistance of water, the amount of energy required to swim a certain distance is greater than that needed to run or walk the same distance. In other words, swimming burns more calories than running or walking.

7. Stationary Cycling/Bicycling

Stationary cycling or bicycling is an excellent form of aerobic exercise when done continuously.

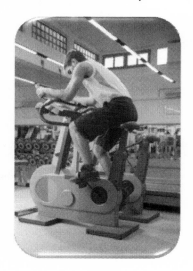

Like swimming, cycling is a non-weight-bearing activity that builds muscular endurance and strength, along with improved flexibility of selected muscles of the legs and thighs.

8. Jumping Rope

Jumping rope can be a great aerobic workout as long as it is performed at a slow to moderate pace and is done continuously for a relatively long period of time (such as 15 minutes).

The key to effective weight loss is through the use of a healthy exercise program that is performed on a regular basis while following a healthy diet & nutritional plan. Aerobic exercise is good for weight loss because it uses more calories than other activities and helps raise your metabolic rate, which helps your body burn calories at a faster rate. It is an effective way to lose fat, but only if you are motivated enough to workout frequently. Aerobics only burns fat during the workout, so if you want encouraging results, you need to be able to exercise daily and for longer periods.

Cardiovascular Exercises

Cardio exercise is one of the best ways to burn a lot of calories while losing extra body fat and giving your metabolism a big boost. Cardio exercises are those that raise your heart rate to 65-90% of your maximum heart rate.

Cardiovascular fitness is considered to be the most important area of physical fitness. Cardiovascular fitness is based on maximizing oxygen intake. This is best achieved through physical activity involving large muscle groups over prolonged periods of time. These activities are rhythmic and aerobic in nature, such as walking, running, hiking, stair climbing, swimming, cycling, rowing, dancing, skating, cross-country skiing, rope jumping, and many more.

When to do it

The best time to do cardio exercises for maximum fat loss is right away in the morning before you eat anything. After you've been asleep for 6-8 hours, the level of sugar (glucose) in your blood is very low, so your body will use stored fat as an alternative energy source.

Significance

- Increases calorie and fat burn

- Weight loss

- Reduces the risk of heart disease

- Increased lung capacity

- Reduced blood pressure

- Prevents diabetes

- Increase metabolism (see BMR)

- Strengthens the cardiovascular system

- Strengthens the immune system

- Lowers stress levels

Weight Training

Some authorities claim that this is the best fat-burning exercise on the grounds that the metabolism continues to burn at an increased rate for 24 hours after a 60-minute workout. In addition, weight training leads to the development of greater lean muscle mass, because of its ability to utilize calories more efficiently.

It also firms and tones the figure, while combating any muscular wastage that can result from prolonged dieting and, together with aerobic exercise or increased daily activity, helps to boost the body's metabolism when the calorie intake is reduced.

Weight training is usually done at your local gym since they have complete equipment. Plus, there are programs where you can enroll with an instructor to guide you through the right exercises, number of repetitions, and duration of each activity. In such places, professionals will monitor your weight loss and guarantee your safety. On the other hand, if you can afford to buy the right equipment for weight training and workouts, then you could do the activity right inside your house. It is more convenient, and you can exercise whenever you want.

Exercise Tools and Equipments

These exercise tools and equipments are related to weight training and workouts since they cannot be done without the right tools, unlike the previous 4 exercises which need only your body, energy, and presence of mind. Advanced exercising machines include electronic devices that measure your weight before and after you exercise, the amount of calories you burned, time elapsed, and other useful information.

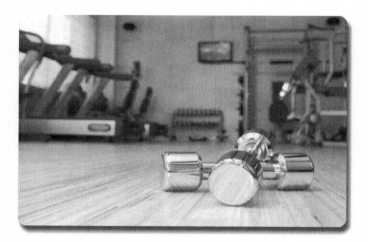

Treadmill

A treadmill is an exercising device consisting of a belt on which a person can walk or jog in place. It is supported by a sturdy deck and propelled either by an electric motor or by the use of the individual. It generally has a shock absorption system and rubber cushioning to minimize stress on your joints.

Using a treadmill will speed up your metabolic rate and allow your body to absorb and utilize a greater quantity of nutrients that you consume. It will also stabilize your insulin levels and blood sugar as well as increase your energy level.

When using a treadmill to lose weight, you need to exercise on a daily basis. A treadmill helps you burn more calories by increasing your exercise frequency. It gives you a LOT of workout versatility. You can start with a slow walk and then speed it up as your body gets into better shape. By using the large muscles of the legs, a treadmill helps you burn major fat calories.

Elliptical Trainer

Elliptical trainers are exercise machines that combine the natural stride of a treadmill with the simplicity of a stair climber. On an elliptical trainer, you stand comfortably in an upright position while holding onto the machine's handrails and striding in either a forward or reverse motion.

The elliptical trainer burns more calories than either the treadmill or the exercise bike. With an elliptical cross trainer, you get the benefits of weight-bearing exercises, such as jogging, without the wear and tear on your joints. It provides a great cardio workout that pumps your heart to the max without the strain and stress on your joints. It uses all of the muscles of the lower leg, therefore, strengthening and building your lower legs. This is an ideal workout for exercisers who are overweight but do not want to jog.

Exercise Bikes

There are two types of exercise bikes you can use: upright bikes and recumbent bikes. Upright bikes simulate the action of a real bike, except you do not go anywhere. Recumbent bikes, on the other hand, have bucket seats and have the pedals out directly in front of you.

Exercise bikes are great for cardiovascular fitness and toning, or building your thighs. The recumbent bikes are especially good for toning your butt. Being that both are stationary, you can enjoy your favorite magazine or TV program while working out.

For overweight people, the bucket seats on recumbent bikes can be more comfortable than traditional uprights. This type of bike is more ergonomically correct than a traditional upright exercise bike and an effective way to improve aerobic capacity, as well as burn fat. Plus, it offers more back support and may be a little more comfortable to those people with lower back pain.

Rowers

There are two types of rowing machines. A hydraulic machine uses a piston to provide resistance. With a cable-driven machine, your movements spin a flywheel, which produces a smooth action similar to rowing on water. The smoothness of the flywheel creates little strain on the back. If the handles are not adjusted properly for height differences, hydraulic rowers can create back strain.

Rowing machines provide a whole-body aerobic workout: arms, shoulders, back, abdomen, legs, heart and lungs. They also build muscle strength and endurance, in addition to the aerobic benefits. They improve your whole cardiovascular system with a low-impact workout. Other benefits include improved flexibility and muscle strengthening in the arms, abdomen, and back. Another advantage is that rowing machines do not cause the pounding on the legs and knees that running does.

Steppers

Steppers are available as simple step-bench systems or as computerized stair steppers. They tone the buttocks, thighs, and hips. These are those areas that have a tendency to "balloon" from too many calories and not enough exercise. Stair-stepper workouts are calorie burners that rank as one of the best cardiovascular exercises for people of all ages and fitness levels.

CHAPTER 5
The Proper Lifestyle: Maintaining it Properly

How you live also affects how much weight you gain and lose. You can't expect to lose weight no matter how long you exercise each day if you keep on eating chocolates and other junk foods, or you behave like a couch potato, sitting in front of the TV set for almost half a day, every day. If your lifestyle is like this, a change is needed. Let us kick those unhealthy habits and start getting rid of fat.

Below are some tips that help in losing weight and burning calories and fat. These simple things that are usually taken for granted will really help you achieve your goal if given complete attention. Making these steps a habit and a part of your everyday life will surely make you realize that you should not have gotten into the bad habits earlier, or you might have not gained those stubborn fats.

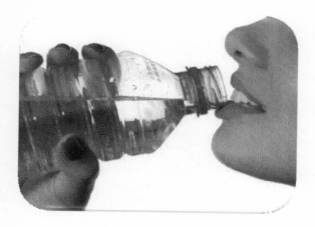

- Drink at least 8 glasses of water every day. This way, you can avoid dehydration, which reduces metabolic rate by 2-3%. Water itself helps cut down on water retention because it acts as a diuretic. When drank before meals, water can dull the appetite as well, so you don't eat as much.

- Eat breakfast. Some in-a-hurry people tend to forget eating early in the morning and just eat more during lunch to make up for it. Eating breakfast raises the metabolic rate by between 10 and 25%, so be sure that you don't skip this important meal.

- Avoid crash-dieting. This lowers the metabolic rate and deprives you of essential nutrients.

- Spread your fat intake over the course of a day. a lot of fat eaten all at once can sharpen the appetite for further fat consumption.

- Stretch your meals to last at least 20 minutes, if not longer. Your stomach, mouth, and brain are all connected, and it takes 20 minutes of chewing before your stomach signals to your brain that you are full. To feel full and successfully lose weight on any weight-loss program, you need to eat each meal slowly, chewing for 20 minutes or longer.

- Drink tea and coffee regularly. Both increase metabolic rate and fat burning.

- Eat those spicy foods you enjoy. They increase your metabolic rate by 25%.

- Don't weigh yourself too often. Use the tape measure and the fit of your clothes to monitor weight-loss progress. Your weight fluctuates constantly, and you can weigh more at night than you did in the morning, so weight is not a good measure of healthfulness.

- Eat a light carbohydrate snack 30 minutes before a meal; it will fill you up quicker so you eat less overall.

- Keep plenty of crunchy foods, like raw vegetables and air-popped fat-free popcorn, on hand. They're high in fibre, making them satisfying and filling.

- Weight loss is easier with a friend. Caring people can help motivate each other to succeed, so team up with a friend to lose more weight.

- Avoid finger foods that are easy to eat in large amounts.

- Avoid consuming large quantities of fattening liquids, which are so easy to overdo.

- Consume <u>nuts</u> only in small portions, as they are composed of up to 50% fat and have a high <u>calorie count</u>.

- Make the kitchen off-limits at any time other than mealtime.

- Always eat at the table, never in front of the TV set or with the radio on. You won't be able to effectively monitor your eating habits when you're enjoying something else at the same time.

- Don't gulp down your food. Savor each bite and concentrate on chewing every mouthful slowly.

- If you're a late-night snacker, eat high-fibre carbs, such as a slice of brown bread or a wholemeal cracker biscuit, before bedtime to cut down on cravings.

- If tempted by a treat, you could eat half and then give the rest away.

- Drink hot water with lemon.

- Eat hot meals rather than cold. Your metabolism speeds up very slightly when you eat, even more so if the food is hot.

- Don't eat anything for the last three or four hours of your day. Once you've had dinner, be done for the night.

- Don't eat anything unnecessary. You don't need "all the fixings".

- Learn to control yourself at social affairs. Don't use them as an excuse to pig out. Be strong.

- Serve yourself normal portions of food. Three ounces of meat or a half cup of rice are plenty in one meal.

- Don't nibble on things throughout the day. Some tidbits contain hundreds of calories.

- Use a smaller plate than usual for dinner. You'll feel like you ate more than you actually did.

- Don't work while eating. Separate all of your activities from your meals, so you can concentrate on what and how much you're eating.

- Don't eat a single bite while preparing meals. Chew gum, if it helps to keep your mouth occupied.

- Never get seconds. Make a habit of stopping after one plate of food.

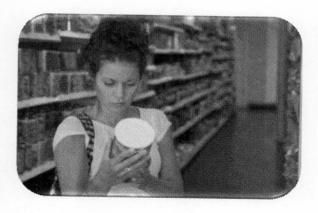

- Put leftovers away immediately to avoid further grazing.

- Read labels carefully. Some low-fat items are very high in calories.

- To slow yourself down, eat with the opposite hand you usually eat with.

- Craving chocolate? Eat a banana. It sometimes satisfies the yearning for chocolate and is much less fattening.

- Chew sugarless gum. It speeds up the digestive system to help you burn more calories, and sometimes it kills a craving too.

- Grab something to drink. Sometimes, cravings for food are really thirst in disguise.

- Exercise – even in school! Take advantage of the gym and PE classes in school. Participate in any sports you can.

- Spend at least 10 minutes per day exercising in your room.

- If possible, walk places instead of riding in a car. You can even enjoy the scenic spots you would miss if you were flying by in a car.

- Use stairs instead of elevators if you're just going up 3-4 stories.

- Limit your TV time to 2 hours or less per day.

- Eat first before strolling at the mall. This way, calories will start burning and at the same time, you won't be tempted to order another burger or french fries.

- Don't shop when you're <u>hungry</u>. You'll only buy more fattening food.

- Substitute activity for junk food. When the cravings hit, walk around the block, do some housework, read, or just do anything just that will take your mind off those old habits.

- Do at least thirty minutes of cardiovascular exercise, five days a week. This will condition you to burn fat more efficiently.

- Wear a pedometer and see that you take 1,000 steps every day.

- If you have a sit-down job, get up every hour and walk around for five minutes or so.

- Dedicate two hours per week to weight training, concentrating on the larger muscles. Every other day is optimal.

- Don't be so hard on yourself. The more positive your self-esteem, the better you feel about yourself, and the faster and easier it will be for you to lose weight. When you are self-confident, you are better able to take charge of your life. It also means that after you lose weight, it will be gone permanently.

- Negative emotions will also interfere with your weight-loss program. It's difficult to stay motivated to lose weight when you feel bad about yourself. Overeating often accompanies negative emotions such as depression, anxiety, fear, guilt, and anger.

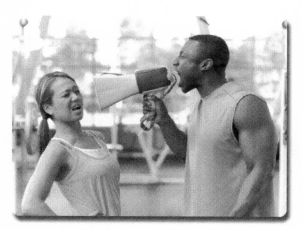

Thus, if you really want to lose weight and burn all the excess body fat away – to be physically fit and healthy – you have to deal with it properly. Proper planning, attitude, diet, exercise, and lifestyle comprise the proper way to achieve your goals. Success is not attained overnight, so you have to really exert not just an effort, but also patience and determination if you want to get thinner and slimmer.

CHAPTER 6
Before And After Transformations

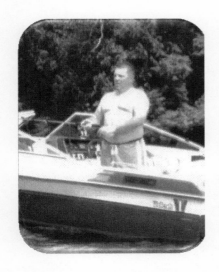

BEFORE

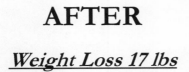

Brian Archer

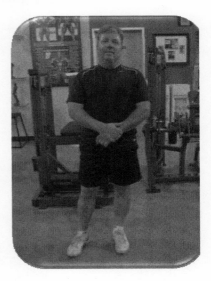

AFTER

Weight Loss 17 lbs

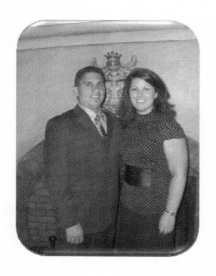

BEFORE

Christinarivera

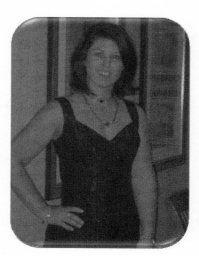

AFTER

Weight Loss 35 lbs

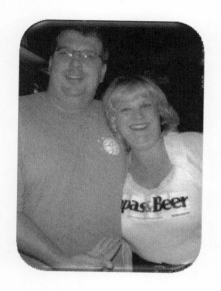

BEFORE

Dave

AFTER

Weight Loss 80 lbs

In 1 year

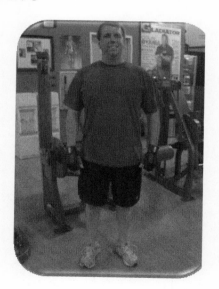

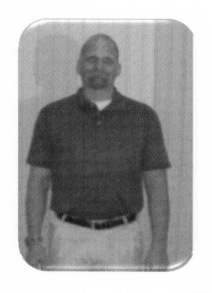

BEFORE

Dave

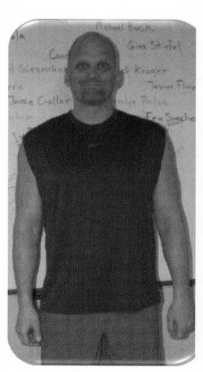

AFTER

Weight Loss 18 lbs

In 6 weeks

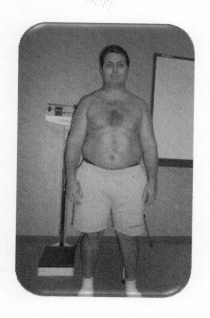

BEFORE

Devin

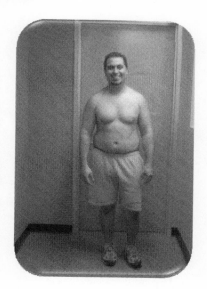

AFTER

Weight Loss 17 lbs

In 6 weeks

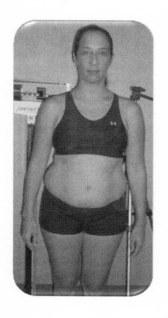

BEFORE

Donna

AFTER

Weight Loss 20 lbs

In 6 weeks

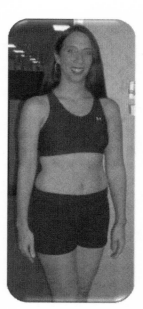

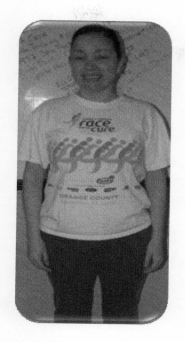

BEFORE

Gabriela

AFTER

Weight Loss 9 lbs

In 6 weeks

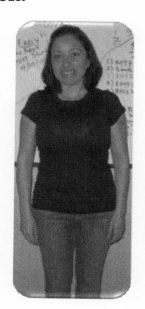

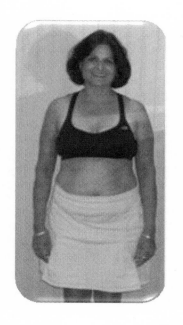

BEFORE

Georgette

AFTER

Weight Loss 15 lbs

In 6 weeks

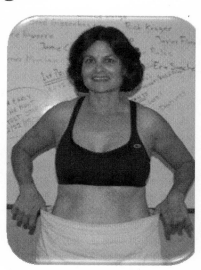

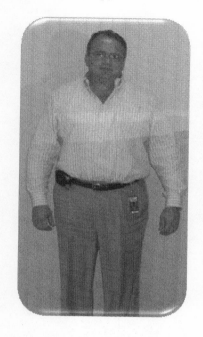

BEFORE

Jim

AFTER

Weight Loss 25 lbs

In 6 weeks

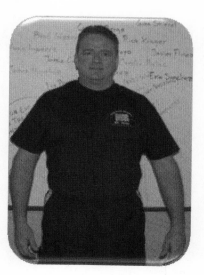

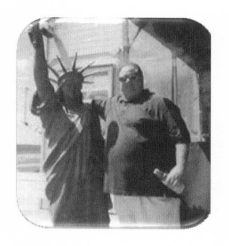

BEFORE

Joeyv

AFTER

Lost over 100 lbs

In one year

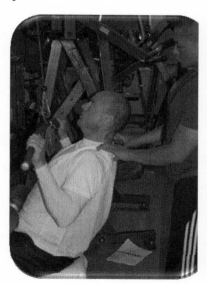

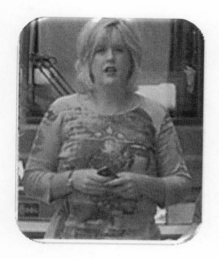

BEFORE

Karen

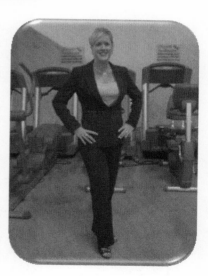

AFTER

Weight Loss 66 lbs
In one year

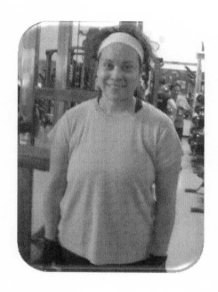

BEFORE

Lillian

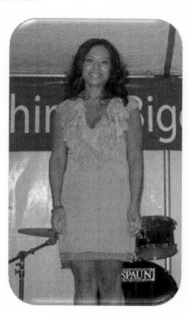

AFTER

Weight Loss 52 lbs

In 7 months

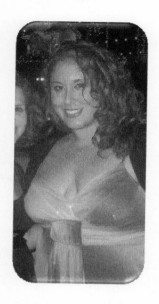

BEFORE

Lisa

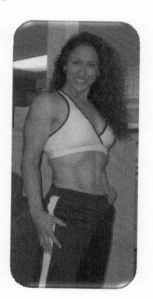

AFTER

Weight Loss 84 lbs

In 9 months

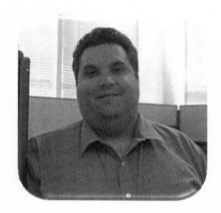

BEFORE

Michael

AFTER

Weight Loss 118 lbs

In one year

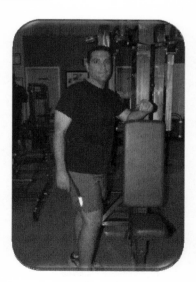

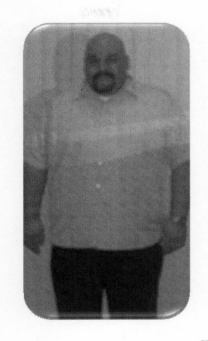

BEFORE

Rob

AFTER

Weight Loss
35 pounds

In 6 weeks

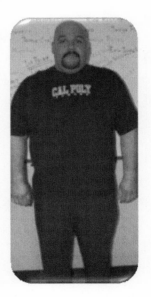

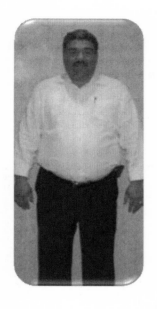

BEFORE

Robert

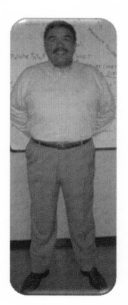

AFTER

Weight Loss
44 pounds

In 6 weeks

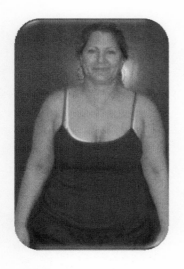

BEFORE

Ronni

AFTER

Weight Loss 23 lbs

In 6 weeks

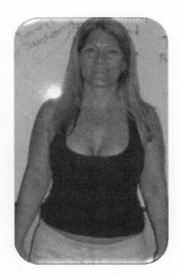

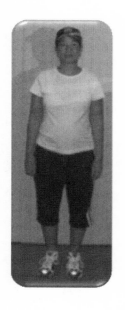

BEFORE

Tamela

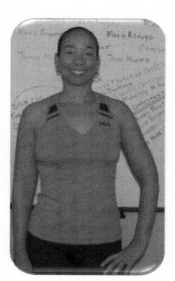

AFTER

Weight Loss 21 lbs

In 6 weeks

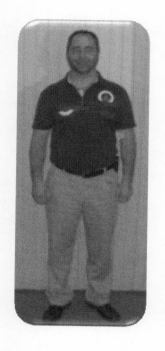

BEFORE

Ted

AFTER

Weight Loss 15 lbs

In 6 weeks

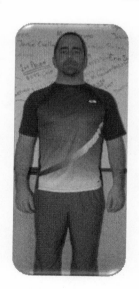

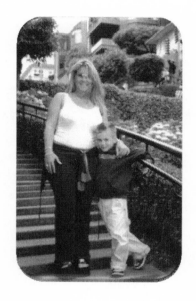

BEFORE

Tiffany

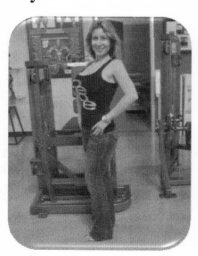

AFTER

Weight Loss 25 lbs

In 4 weeks

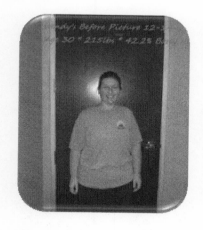

BEFORE

Wendy

AFTER

Weight Loss 16 lbs

In 6 weeks

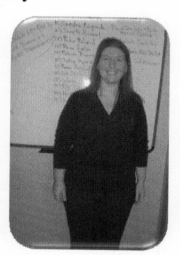

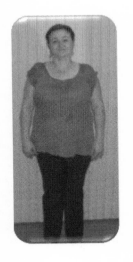

BEFORE

Yesenia

AFTER

Weight Loss 11.5 lbs

In 6 weeks

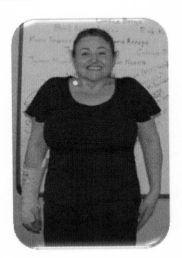

RESOURCES

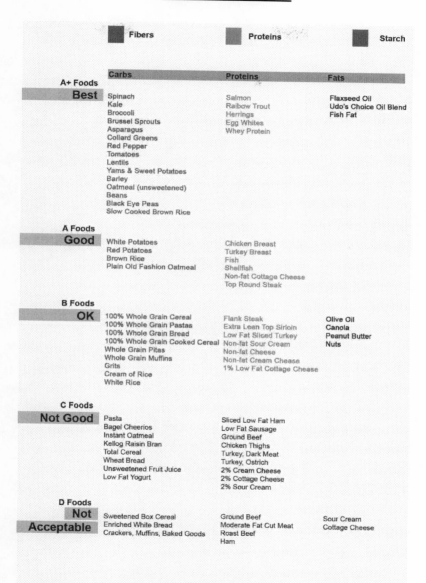

	Fibers		Proteins		Starch

	Carbs	Proteins	Fats
A+ Foods **Best**	Spinach Kale Broccoli Brussel Sprouts Asparagus Collard Greens Red Pepper Tomatoes Lentils Yams & Sweet Potatoes Barley Oatmeal (unsweetened) Beans Black Eye Peas Slow Cooked Brown Rice	Salmon Rainbow Trout Herrings Egg Whites Whey Protein	Flaxseed Oil Udo's Choice Oil Blend Fish Fat
A Foods **Good**	White Potatoes Red Potatoes Brown Rice Plain Old Fashion Oatmeal	Chicken Breast Turkey Breast Fish Shellfish Non-fat Cottage Cheese Top Round Steak	
B Foods **OK**	100% Whole Grain Cereal 100% Whole Grain Pastas 100% Whole Grain Bread 100% Whole Grain Cooked Cereal Whole Grain Pitas Whole Grain Muffins Grits Cream of Rice White Rice	Flank Steak Extra Lean Top Sirloin Low Fat Sliced Turkey Non-fat Sour Cream Non-fat Cheese Non-fat Cream Cheese 1% Low Fat Cottage Cheese	Olive Oil Canola Peanut Butter Nuts
C Foods **Not Good**	Pasta Bagel Cheerios Instant Oatmeal Kellog Raisin Bran Total Cereal Wheat Bread Unsweetened Fruit Juice Low Fat Yogurt	Sliced Low Fat Ham Low Fat Sausage Ground Beef Chicken Thighs Turkey, Dark Meat Turkey, Ostrich 2% Cream Cheese 2% Cottage Cheese 2% Sour Cream	
D Foods **Not** **Acceptable**	Sweetened Box Cereal Enriched White Bread Crackers, Muffins, Baked Goods	Ground Beef Moderate Fat Cut Meat Roast Beef Ham	Sour Cream Cottage Cheese

F Grade foods include 1) trans fats, 2) foods in high saturated fats, 3) highly processed or refined foods, 4) highly sweetened foods or foods that are pure sugar, 5) foods that are high in refined sugars and fats, 6) processed, high fat meats.

Note: Fruits are very good for you but must be limited on a fat loss diet. One or two fruits/day are recommended.

Recommended Beverages

Water	*Try to drink at least 64 ounces of water per day (nothing beats mother nature)*
Crystal Light or Flavored Water	*Great way to drink more water with adding a little flavor to it.*
Diet Soda	*Not good for your health, however if you are craving something sweet it can help without providing calories.*
Coffee	*Caffeine is a natural fat burner. Black coffee in moderation helps burn fat. Although drinking too much will dehydrate you.*
100% Juice	*Although it contains a lot of sugar and calories (which is not good when trying to lose weight), it is a great source of vitamins & antioxidants when trying to maintain weught.*
Tea	*Unsweetened green tea is a very good source of antioxidants.*

Recommended Condiments

Salsa

Yeloow or Dijon Mustard

Fat Free Dressing/Spritz

Ketchup*

Balsamic Vinegar

Hot Sauces

Butter Spray*

Meal 1	Time

Meal 2	Time

Meal 3	Time

Meal 4	Time

Meal 5	Time

Meal 6	Time

Fat Fighting Tips

• Do Aerobics in the Morning

Scientific studies show doing aerobic exercises for about 20 minutes, first thing in the morning, could be more effective for burning fat than a full hour of aerobic exercise later in the day after you've eaten a few meals. You see, after an overnight fast, blood sugar levels are low, as are carbohydrate reserves. Exercising before you eat causes the body to dip right into storedfat to come up with the necessary energy required to make it through whatever rude awakening you've subjected it to.

• Don't Starve Yourself

Reducing your calorie intake to an amount less than 8 times your body weight may cause your metabolism to institute sever energy-saving measures that will make you dim-witted and grumpy, as well as reduce the rate your body burns calories. It may also cause a reduction in lean body mass or muscle. By feeding your body frequently (up to 6 times) throughout the day, you can avoid hunger cramps and maintain stable energy levels and a healthy metabolism.

• Build More Muscle

Muscle has a twofold cosmetic function. It not only helps you look healthier and stronger but it also makes your bore metabolically active. Muscle burns calories even while you are sitting there, but fat is metabolically inactive. The more muscle you have the more calories you need just to maintain your present weight. So, if you build muscle, you can eat more and not gain weight.

• Consume More Protein

A gram of fat contains roughly 9 calories while a gram of carbohydrates or protein contains just 4. For years, dietitians and scientists alike assumed one calorie was pretty much like another, and if you eat too many of them, they'd all end up being stored fat. It turns out that's not necessarily true. Studies show if you eat 100 calories of carbs, it takes the body about 23 calories just to process it. The energy "cost" to digest protein is even higher. However, if you eat 100 calories of fat, it takes the body just 3 calories to process and deposit it.

• Count "Portions", not Calories

There aren't many people who can keep track of their calorie intake for an extended period of time. As an alternative, I recommend count "portions". A portion of food is roughly equal to the size of your clenched fist, or the palm of your hand. Each portion of protein or carbs typically contains between 100 and 150 calories. For example, one chicken breast is approximately one portion of protein, and one medium sized baked potato is approximately one portion of carbs.

• Caffeine May Help Burn Fat

Supplements like Phen-Free, which contain caffeine, used 30 to 60 minutes before and aerobic workout, may allow you to burn fat faster. In scientific studies, caffeine has been shown to help liberate fatty acids from body fat stores, thus possibly increasing your body's ability to burn fat. It may also increase strength and focus during a workout and is often used for this purpose.

• Cut Back on Carbs at Night

It's a scientific fact that your body cannot burn fat while your insulin levels are elevated. It's also a fact that carbs cause insulin to go up. So, it's especially important to limit your carb intake of foods like bread, pasta, potatoes, rice, candy, juice, crackers, and bagels in the evening around 6:00 p.m. Carbs consumed in the evening are more likely to be converted to body fat and/or reduce the amount of fat your body may burn during sleep.

• "Pig Out" Once a Week

No one can eat "perfectly" all the time without going crazy! If you are craving something like apple pie, French fries, pizza or candy, hold off that craving until your "free day". One day a week, forget calorie counting, portion control, etc. and eat whatever you'd like. By giving yourself this option, you can maintain the discipline you need to be successful the other six days of the week.

• Don't Just Read These Tips – Follow Them!

Fibers   **Proteins**   **Starch**

Grocery Store
Shopping List

Proteins:
- Boneless Skinless Chicken
- Turkey Breast
- Lean Red Meats
  - Flank Steak
  - London Broil
  - Top Cirloin
  - 4% Ground Beef
- Fish
  - Tuna
  - Halibut
  - Tilapia
  - Mahi Mahi
  - Red Snapper
  - Shark Steak
  - Salmon*
- Egg Whites

Good Fats
- Almonds
- Peanuts
- Flaxseed and Olive Oil
- Peanut Butter
- Avocados
- Pam and utter Spray (Alternative to oil/butter)

Poly Un-saturated fat
- Safflower
- Sunflower
- Soybean
- Corn
- Cottonseed

Mono Un-saturated Fat
- Olive Oil
- Canola Oil
- Peanut Oil
- Avocados

Dairy
- 2% Non-fat Cottage Cheese
- Damon Light & Fit Yogurt
- Fat Free Milk*

Complex/Starchy Carbohydrates
- Grits
- Oatmeal
- Red potatoes
- Yams
- Brown/White Rice*
- Whole Wheat Pasta
- Whole Wheat Bread
- Cream of Wheat

Fibrous Carbohydrates
- Broccoli
- Asparagus
- Spinach
- Green Beans
- Brussel Sprouts
- Cabbage
- Cauliflower
- Zucchini
- Onions
- Tomatoes
- Mushrooms
- Squash
- Eggplants
- Alfalfa
- Bock Choy
- Cucumber
- Lettuce
- Artichokes

Things to keep in mind: 1) Complex/Starchy carbs are good for long-term energy, so plan to eat these according to your day's activities. **2) Fibrous carbs** are the best for getting lean. It makes you feel full without providing many calories. 3) even though **"good fats"** are good for you they still provide a 9 kcal/gram, so limit when trying to get lean. **4) Poly un-saturated fat** is found mostly from plant sources, which tend to lower your cholesterol level. **5) Mon un-saturated fat** tend to lower LDL "bad cholesterol", found in animal and plant products. **6) Saturated "bad" fat** tend to increase cholesterol level and most are solid at room temperature (except tropicals oils). Butter is also high in saturated fat.

Resistance Training

Exercise	Seat Adj.	Set 1		Set 2		Set 3		Set 4	
		Wt	Rep	Wt	Rep	Wt	Rep	Wt	Rep
1									
2									
3									
4									
5									
6									
7									
8									
9									
10									
11									
12									
13									

Food Supplementation

Workout Supplements	Dosage	Before Workout	After Workout

Cardiovascular Program

Mode		Program	
Time		Level	

NOTES

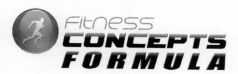

14682 Central Ave., Chino, CA 91710

<u>NOTES</u>

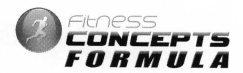

<u>14682 Central Ave., Chino, CA 91710</u>

NOTES

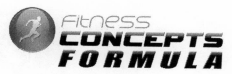

14682 Central Ave., Chino, CA 91710

NOTES

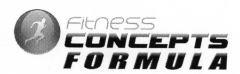

14682 Central Ave., Chino, CA 91710

<u>NOTES</u>

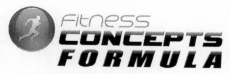

<u>14682 Central Ave., Chino, CA 91710</u>

NOTES

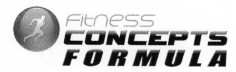

14682 Central Ave., Chino, CA 91710

NOTES

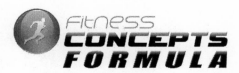

14682 Central Ave., Chino, CA 91710

NOTES

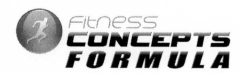

14682 Central Ave., Chino, CA 91710

APPENDIX A
Desirable Weight Ranges

Males		Females	
HEIGHT	WEIGHT	HEIGHT	WEIGHT
5'4"	117 - 163	5'0"	96 - 138
5'5"	120 - 167	5'1"	99 - 141
5'6"	124 - 173	5'2"	102 - 144
5'7"	128 - 178	5'3"	105 - 149
5'8"	132 - 183	5'4"	108 - 152
5'9"	136 - 187	5'5"	111 - 156
5'10"	140 - 193	5'6"	114 - 161
5'11"	144 - 198	5'7"	118 - 165
6'0"	148 - 204	5'8"	122 - 169
6'1"	152 - 209	5'9"	126 - 174
6'2"	156 - 215	5'10"	130 - 179
6'3"	160 - 220	5'11"	134 - 185
6'4"	169 - 231	6'0"	138 - 190

APPENDIX B
Food Calorie Table

Calorie Table for Breakfast Cereal Food	Calorie Content
Corn Flakes, Kelloggs	(45 g) 167
Rice Krispies, Kelloggs	(45 g) 171
Corn flakes, regular	(1 cup) 110
Calorie Table for Bread and Bakery	**Calorie Content**
Biscuit (15 g)	74
White Bread (1 slice/37 g)	84
Danish Pastry	287
Doughnut (49 g)	140
Hot Cross Bun (70 g)	205
Calorie Table for Eggs and Dairy	**Calorie Content**
Butter (10 g)	74
Cheese, Cheddar (40 g)	172
Eggs, whole (extra large/58 g)	86
Egg, white (large)	16
Egg, yolk (large)	59
Buffalo milk (1 cup)	17
Calories in milk, semi skimmed (200ml)	96
Calorie Table for Fruits	**Calorie Content**
Apple (112g)	53
Banana (150g)	143
Grapes (50g)	30
Melon (1oz/28g)	7
Orange (160g)	59
Pear (170g)	68
Strawberries (1oz/28g)	7
Calorie Table for Vegetables	**Calorie Content**
Carrots (60g)	13
Peas (60g)	32
Salad (100g)	19
Broccoli (4 oz)	15
Cabbage, raw (1 cup)	25

Cauliflower, raw (1 cup)	30
Onions (4 oz)	40
Mushrooms (1 cup)	18
Potato, sweet (4 oz)	80
Potatoes, baked (4 oz)	104
Potatoes, boiled (4 oz)	80
Radishes (4 oz)	15
Spinach (1 cup)	10
Tomato (medium)	20
Calorie Table for Meat and Chicken	**Calorie Content**
Bacon (1 Rasher/25g)	64
Chicken breast (200g)	342
Beef, gravy (83 ml)	45
Ham, 1 slice (30g)	35
Kebab (168g)	429
Calorie Table for Chocolates and Sweets	**Calorie Content**
Chocolate (100g)	530
Chocolate ice cream (50g)	159
Mars Bar (65g)	294
Popcorn (100g)	405
Low-calorie sweetener (1 tsp/1g)	4
Chewing gum, Wrigley's (1 piece)	10
Calorie Table for Drinks	**Calorie Content**
Coffee (1 cup/220 ml)	154
Can of Coke (330 ml)	139
Orange Juice (1 glass/200 ml)	88
Tea (1 mug/270 ml)	29
Chocolate shake (generic) (10 oz)	360
Calorie table for Fast Food	**Calorie Content**
Big Mac (215g)	492
Kentucky Fried Chicken (67g)	195
Hamburger (108g)	254
Pizza (½ pizza/135g)	263
McDonald's French Fries (small)	210

APPENDIX C
Calories Burned During Exercises
(and other activities)

ACTIVITY	CALORIES/HOUR
Bowling	250
Cleaning windows	350
Cycling	400
Dancing	300
Football	450
Gardening	250
General housework	190
Golf	250
Horse riding	450
Ironing	250
Jogging	500
Mowing the lawn	400
Running	900
Scrubbing floors	275
Skiing	500
Swimming	500
Walking	250

SUMMARY

The real richness in life, more than money and property, is living a healthy life – without concerns that certain illnesses might attack us. Unlike material things that come and go, our health is something that we can invest in while we are still young and use until we grow old. Thus, we should take good care of it and never take it for granted.

Our weight is one basis of measuring if we are healthy or not – whether we belong to the category of underweight, normal, overweight, or obese. There are two ways of knowing where we belong: through the common height-weight relationship and through our body mass index (BMI). Either way, one has to know if he is healthy or not in order to make certain adjustments, or, in the worst-case scenario, treatments.

Obesity, defined as being 20 percent or more above one's desirable weight range, is a serious illness that should not be left untreated as it can bring serious health complications. According to studies, obesity may be caused by genetic factors, i.e. if any of the family members, especially the parents, suffer from such sickness, the children will most likely inherit it from them. The same can be true with improper eating habits and/or lifestyle. Effects of obesity include both psychological and biological aspects like heart diseases, cancer, diabetes, and much more. Thus, if obesity can't be terminated immediately, who knows what could happen next? The ending of one's life is not an impossible effect, unfortunately.

Luckily, it's not yet too late. Obesity, indeed, can be be cured…and even prevented. All it takes is a "proper" way of dealing with it, plus patience, determination, and will. And before you know it, your weight might have decreased by 20 pounds or your waistline trimmed down by 10 inches. Isn't that cool? Not to mention healthy!

So, what's the proper way to lose weight? The proper way is actually just altering your everyday lifestyle and habits. First, you've got to have a proper plan. This includes setting a goal of what you want to accomplish in a certain period of time. It should be definite and realistic. Strategizing in an organized manner is part of the plan. Time and duration of activities to be done throughout the day or week should be noted and remembered. Positive thinking and the right attitude towards weight loss are also important in making plans work. Believing that something will happen triggers the body to do things that could make your hopes and dreams come true. Thus, although plans are still in your mind and not yet turning into reality, they are a good help in starting to make things happen.

Eating is the habit most associated with body weight and obesity. Everyone eats…but not everyone does it properly. Proper diet should contain all food nutrients, such as carbohydrates, proteins, vitamins, and minerals, making your meal healthy and nutritious. In contrast to what most people believe, all fats are not bad for our body. In fact, there are good fats, such as unsaturated fats, and their intake should not be limited. The unhealthy fats are those that belong to the saturated group of fats.

Since obesity is related to heavier weight and excess body fat, weight loss with regards to food intake involves either one of two ways: eating low-fat foods, or consuming fat-burning foods. The former diet is about substituting high-fat foods for those with low-fat contents, while the latter refers to simply eating foods that burn excess fats in the body. Either of those diets will surely help you lose weight and get rid of those stubborn body fats.

Losing weight is not dependent on the right diet alone, however. To speed it up and burn more calories faster, one should engage in proper exercises, which include deep breathing, walking, aerobic exercises, cardiovaslcular exercises, and weight training. Also, there are exercise machines and tools that can help you lose weight, such as treadmills, exercise bikes, steppers, and many more.

Lastly, one should also watch his lifestyle if he really wants to cure his illness and, eventually, maintain his weight correctly. Proper lifestyle, although composed of simple and little everyday things, will really affect a lot in reducing weight. Thus, one should not take his habits for granted, even those that are as trivial as eating in front of the TV or choosing the best time to go shopping.

CONCLUSION

So, you think you're ready to lose weight and burn fat? To motivate you even more, remember that it's not just your heavy weight and your stubborn body fat that you can eliminate with these proper guidelines, but also a really dangerous illness that may be fatal – obesity.

Obesity is a killer. It does not do any good…only harm to innocent people like you and me. It's worse than criminals that try to attack us. Bad people can be seen and known in the surroundings. We can try to avoid them or fight against them when encountered. There are powerful authorities that ostracize them when caught and give them the right punishment according to how badly they behaved. But obesity is far different from lawbreakers. Although both may slay us, obesity kills without the victim knowing it. When it gets complicated and serious, there can be no escape.

Obesity poisons both our body and mind. For the former, its weapon is an overload of fats targetting essential body parts and organs, thus bringing serious complications like heart diseases, cancer, stomach problems, and a lot more. As for the latter, negative thinking often goes hand in hand with obesity, making the victim feel inferior and underrated among other people around him.

Terrible, isn't it? So before it becomes too late, before it attacks us and bring us down to our last breath, why don't we counter its assault? Let us be the ones who terminate obesity first before it kills us. There's nothing and nobody else that can help us completely but ourselves.

Perhaps that is the reason why the world has no place for obesity – because it kills. Well, then, show the world that you can terminate what they have been rejecting all the while. Let them notice you, see you, and recognize you the way you really should be seen…as a person, not just a statistic. ☺

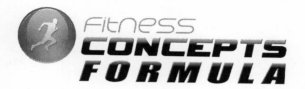

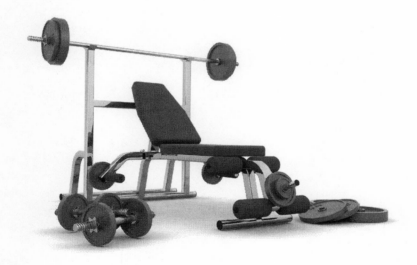

www.fitconcepts.com

Thank you very much for choosing Fitness Concepts for your fitness needs. Our goal is to provide you with excellent service throughout our program. We are committed to provide our clients with knowledge, tools, and motivation to succeed in their quest for fitness and health. Since 1999, we have helped thousands of our clients get in the best shape of their life and we want to do the same for you.

Committed to your fitness success:
Saman Bakhtiar
Owner

P.S. Please feel free to contact me anytime if there are any questions and/or concerns you may have. We are always looking to better serve our clients. I can be reached at (909) 693-5287 or email at Sam@fitconcepts.com

Resources

www.FitnessGuruSam.com
www.AskDoctorSam.com
www.Facebook.com/FitnessConcepts
www.FitConceptsInnerCircle.com

76650398R00121

Made in the USA
Columbia, SC
25 September 2019